DENTAL IMPLANT TREATMENT PLANNING

FOR NEW DENTISTS STARTING IMPLANT THERAPY

Dr. Nkem Obiechina

Images of Implant Restorations from Dr. Dalvir Pannu and Pannu Dental Associates

AuthorHouse™
1663 Liberty Drive
Bloomington, IN 47403
www.authorhouse.com
Phone: 833-262-8899

Published by AuthorHouse   02/04/2022

ISBN: 978-1-5462-2111-1 (sc)
ISBN: 978-1-5462-2110-4 (e)

Library of Congress Control Number: 2017919107

Illustrated By: Alex Stone Illustrator

Print information available on the last page.

Any people depicted in stock imagery provided by Thinkstock are models, and such images are being used for illustrative purposes only. Certain stock imagery © Thinkstock.

This book is printed on acid-free paper.

authorHOUSE®

Contents

Introduction v

Chapter 1: Implant Treatment planning.. 1

Chapter 2: Assessment of conditions that can affect dental implant placement............................. 15

Chapter 3: Dental Implant Components and Protocols for Dental Implant surgery 22

Chapter 4: Late, Early and Immediate implant placement.. 30

Chapter 5: Site preparation prior and during Dental Implant placement. 40

Chapter 6: Bone and Soft tissue augmentation procedures prior to dental Implant placement 45

Chapter 7: Preparation and Steps for Dental Implant Surgery. 48

Chapter 8: Dental Implant Uncovering and Second Stage Implant Surgery............................... 58

Chapter 9: Selecting Dental Implant abutments and Impression techniques for Fixed Implant
           Restorations. 61

Chapter 10: Cemented versus Screw retained dental implant restorations.................................... 69

Chapter 11: Restorative Options for Edentulous patients (Overdentures and Fixed Restorations)....... 72

Chapter 12: Dental Implant Complications 79

Chapter 13: Dental Implant Maintenance.. 84

Chapter 14: Conclusion 89

References 91

Introduction

Dental implants have been one of the most revolutionary discoveries in dentistry changing how dentists view replacement of missing teeth. They have also brought to the forefront other dynamics that have paramount importance in replacing teeth including relationships of the replaced restorations to adjacent teeth and supporting structures such as bone, connective tissue and gingival tissue.

The goal of this book is to offer the new implant dentist with a comprehensive guide to decision making during implant therapy as well as address relevant topics that can be important to dental implant placement and restoration. It also reviews the latest advancements in dental implant therapy with information from current studies on overall success rates in order to offer a valuable resource to a dentist starting to place and restore implants.

Dental implants have afforded dentists the opportunity of offering their patients tooth replacements that are fixed in the mouth without affecting adjacent teeth. They are functionally and esthetically pleasing for patients as well as very comfortable, and require minimum chair time compared to other restorative options such as removable prosthesis that involve multiple appointments for adjustments and relines. As a dentist that has made the decision to implement implant dentistry as part of your dental practice you are making a wise choice.

Over the past 30-40 years, there has been a major increase in the number of dentists placing and restoring dental implants. Implant placement has no longer been designated to periodontists and oral surgeons only, but more general dentists are placing and restoring routine dental implant cases while referring more complicated implant cases.

Implant companies have also teamed up with dentists that use their dental implant systems to offer hands on courses that allow dentists that are new to dental implants to place implants into study models or mandibles of animals. The goal of their implant courses has been to provide hands on experience on the implant procedure for dentists prior to their implementing surgical and implant restoration procedures at their practices. In addition, multiple seminars and webinars are available with videos and live courses that show surgical placement and restoration of dental implants on patients.

The general consensus is that despite receiving prior training from these courses and from various other sources, when it is time to offer dental implants as part of dental practice, most dentists encounter challenges as they gain the necessary experience that they require to fully implement dental implants as part of their daily practice.

The goal of this book is to provide a guide to treatment planning and placement of dental implants for new dentists who are implementing dental implants as part of their dental practice, as well as provide some practical answers to some questions that they might have during the initial process. It is also our goal to draw from the latest studies in order to provide dentists with as much information possible prior to implementing dental implants. The beginning of the book starts as a preview of dental implant planning, while the remainder of book is divided into two sections, one dealing with surgical dental implant placement, the other section dealing with dental implant restoration.

During dental implant treatment planning key decisions have to be made which can involve the type of surgical protocol to choose, whether to choose a one stage, non-submerged implant placement, versus two stage implant surgical technique involving a submerged dental implant protocol. Decisions on whether to use CT guided technology or non guided surgery, as well as if a flapless technique or mucoperiosteal flap will be utilized for surgery are all decisions that should be made prior to the dental implant surgery. They will be reviewed in detail in the book so that pertinent information is available when making the choice. Anatomic and local factors related to the implant site as well as location of the implant site in the mouth also affect dental implant treatment planning and will be reviewed also.

The planning phase also involves other decisions such as what type of temporary restoration to utilize during osteo-integration, or whether bone or soft tissue grafting would be needed before dental implant placement and what type of bone graft and soft tissue graft would be necessary. Anatomic, functional and esthetic factors affecting dental implant placement all have to be understood in the treatment planning stage and will be also reviewed as well in this book.

For dentists that are interested in restoring dental implants a number of choices are available and therefore we will review guidelines in choosing types of abutments. Options include custom versus standard, zircornia versus metal abutments, angled versus straight abutments. Also, how to choose the optimal abutment height during dental implant restoration will also be reviewed. The use of cemented versus screw retained restorations will also be reviewed in detail, and understanding the rationale behind choosing various dental implant components as well as the technique to utilize would be important to help ensure success of dental implant placement and restoration.

CHAPTER 1

Implant Treatment planning

In planning dental implants the first step is deciding which patients would be good candidates for implant therapy. The medical history for patients are first reviewed to identify any uncontrolled systemic conditions that can be able to affect dental implant placement. Next, to select the right patient cases, a comprehensive exam involving a clinical exam and radiographic exam utilizing full mouth x-rays and panorex are completed. CT Scans should also be obtained if necessary to view vital structures or for more comprehensive treatment planning especially with multiple implants.

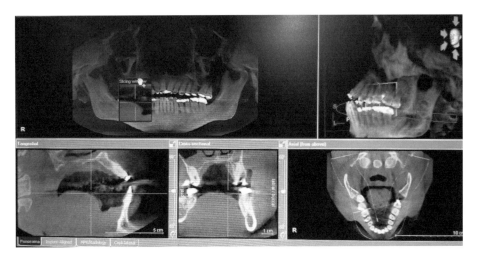

CT Scan showing Panoramic, Crosssectional and Cephalometric views of the mouth

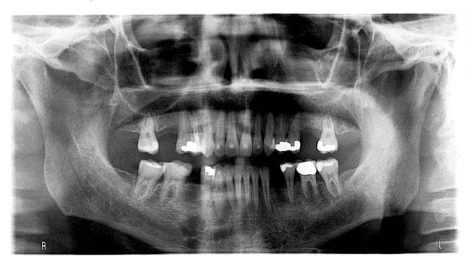

Panorex showing location of inferior alveolar nerve and maxillary sinus

Typically, for single teeth replacements around premolars and molars, Panoramic x-rays to evaluate vital structures such as the maxillary sinus, mental foramen and inferior alveolar nerve are necessary. Peri-apical x-rays can provide a focused view of the implant site. CT Scans can also be utilized to give a better understanding about the bone height, density and width, as well as to allow the anatomy in the area to be visualized. These scans give a three dimensional view of the bone in the implant site and are essential for treatment planning especially for more complex dental implant cases. CT scan imaging does offer a number of advantages even with single tooth dental implant placement by giving a better preoperative visualization of the bone in the dental implant site prior to dental implant placement.

A preliminary dental implant examination allows for assessment of the patient's oral condition, so that all teeth that should be treatment planned for dental implants can be readily visualized. It will also allow the ability to evaluate other teeth in the mouth so that the appropriate restorative options can be chosen, and disease conditions that might hamper the success rate of dental implants can be identified and treated prior to dental implant therapy.

The overall benefit that can be gained from this examination is also that it helps develop a comprehensive course of action that incorporates all treatment needs of a patient during the treatment planning phase. Inter-occlusal and inter-arch space can be evaluated, condition of adjacent teeth, as well as other treatment needs of the patient can also be identified.

The need for periodontics, restorative, prosthodontics, orthodontics, endodontics, and oral surgery is also determined, and the sequence to start therapy is decided. Examination starting from a periodontal evaluation, occlusal analysis, endodontic, and restorative planning should be completed prior to dental implant therapy. Orthodontic assessment and therapy should be completed if needed prior to initiating dental implant therapy unless otherwise recommended by an orthodontist.

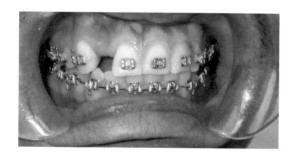
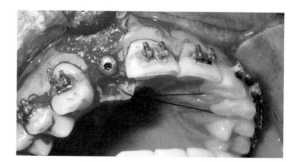
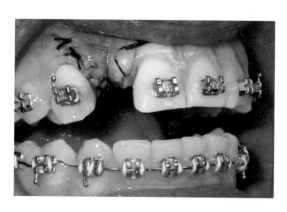
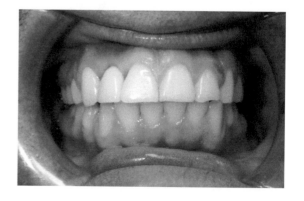

For example, if a patient needs or still has braces on their teeth to correct for extensive spacing or crowding in the arch, collaboration should occur between treating dentists to determine when and where would be ideal to place the dental implant. In addressing spatial concerns, a team approach to dental implant placement is recommended. The team usually comprises orthodontists, implant surgeons and restorative dentists who make decisions about when and where to place the dental implants. Spatial deficiencies and diastemas can be corrected using orthodontics, enamelplasty or restorations prior to placement and restoration of dental implants.[1]

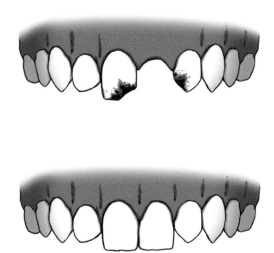

Restoration of caries and other dental conditions needed prior to dental implant placement

Preliminary Dental Implant Examination:

During the initial dental implant assessment, comprehensive restorative and periodontal examinations are completed to assess the condition of adjacent teeth and screen for dental diseases and other pre-existing conditions.

The approach to dental implants especially in the anterior zone is now more of a restoration driven dental implant placement rather than a surgical guided one with dental implants placed in sites that allow the most optimal restorative outcome rather than an emphasis on only where there is adequate bone for implant placement.[1] As a result, the goal of the current approach is to utilize additional techniques such as bone augmentation in other to create more favorable sites for dental implant placement rather than placing implants in situations that present possible restorative complications.

This is particularly important especially when treatment planning and restoring anterior dental implants. A multi-disciplinary approach to dental implant placement is often the goal. If potential complications such as deficient space or inter arch distance, crowding, staining, wear, or caries in adjacent teeth, they should be addressed, and periodontal and endodontic disease that are detected in adjacent teeth should be noted and treated. These conditions when noted during treatment planning are treated by the general dentist if within scope of care, or referred to specialists as needed.

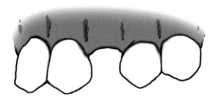

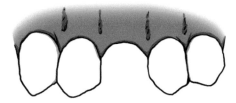

*Inadequate versus adequate
space for dental implants*

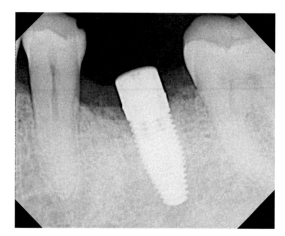

*showing adequate space
for molar crown*

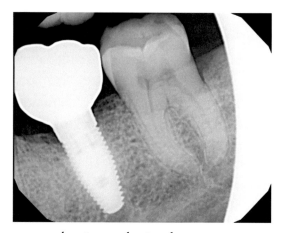

showing molar implant crown

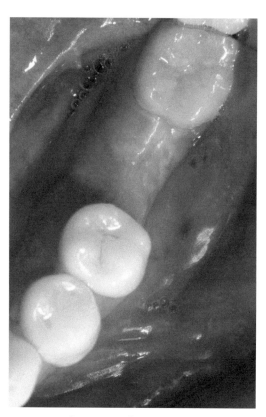

*showing adequate space
for molar implant*

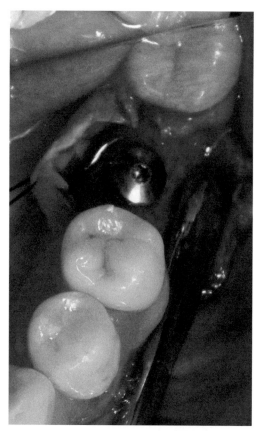

*implant placement with
adequate space*

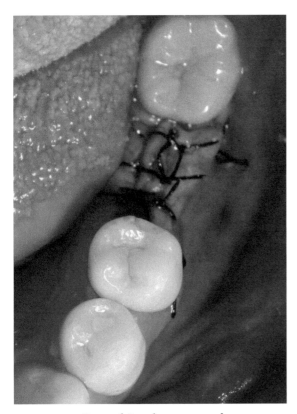

Dental Implant sutured

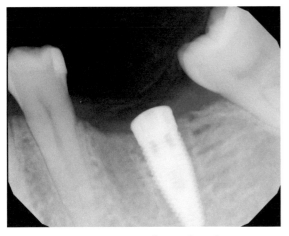

Posterior implant placed

As a dentist that is starting to place dental implants, recommendation is usually made to start placement in the areas of the mouth typically not in the esthetic zone but still accessible such as mandibular and maxillary premolar areas, as well as first molar areas for first implant placement. [2] As level of expertise increases, the anterior zone becomes a viable area for dental implant placement and restoration. However, if your first implant surgery is in the anterior zone, with careful dental implant planning and therapy, you can still be able to get a successful result.

SEQUENCE OF DENTAL IMPLANT TREATMENT PLANNING:

As part of the preliminary examination, impressions for study models are made, allowing fabrication of a diagnostic wax-up by a dental laboratory. This will allow for visualization of potential end results, and provide a guide for achieving successful esthetic outcomes. This can also provide a stent if Ct guided stent is not being utilized.

Specifically, the potential size of the planned implant restoration can be visualized with the wax up, allowing the dentist to evaluate if there is adequate or excessive amount of space for the implants that are treatment planned. It will also allow the dentist to evaluate the potential length of the restoration in comparison to adjacent teeth especially for teeth that have been extracted for a number of years. They can be able to provide guidance such as whether increasing the ridge height or width would be needed and referral for block or particulate bone grafting is needed prior to implant placement. Usually alginate impressions can be taken for preliminary study casts as well as a bite registration which is also provided to the dental lab, for more complex cases a face bow transfer and models mounted on semi adjustable articulators are needed.

The diagnostic wax up would also be a good guide for determining the best restorative option for patients. For example, if the patient would be better served with over dentures versus fixed prosthetic restorations on the implants due to loss of bone and supporting tissues. The wax up would give a guide of the potential optimal option so that a choice can be made to ensure the right restoration is utilized. It will also allow decisions such as whether single implant restorations or splinted implant bridges would be the better option when multiple implants are being placed.

The articulated diagnostic wax up also allows dentists to be able to choose abutments based on the inter-occlusal space present, and assess whether angled abutments, custom or standard abutment would be necessary. The diagnostic wax-up can also be utilized to fabricate temporary restorations as well as provide a template for a surgical guide for dental implant placement.

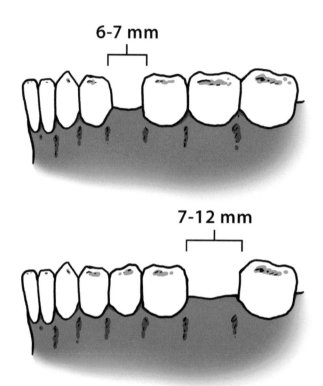

Dimensions for dental implant diameter for premolar and molar sites

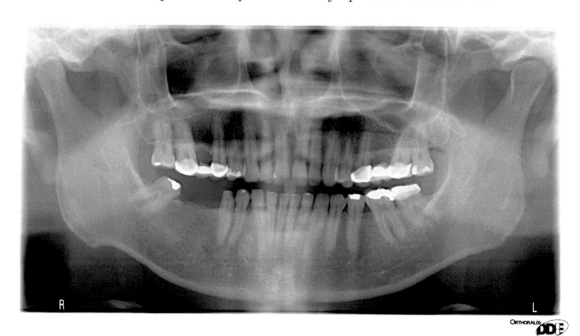

Panorex x-ray showing site that has two missing molars

6

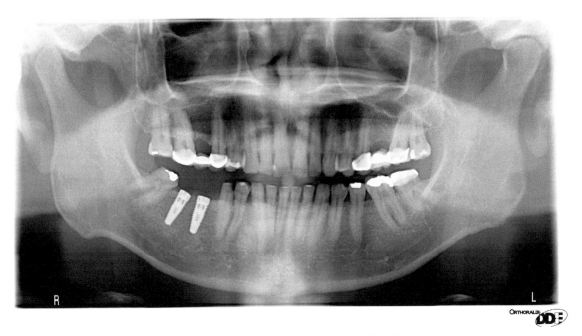

Mandibular dental implants placed

Surgical guides aid in restoration driven dental implant placement. These guides allow the placement of dental implants in optimal positions, not just based on the anatomic characteristics of the bone, but they also in positions that allow cosmetic restorative outcomes. They also facilitate optimal positioning and angulation of implants in bone.[3]

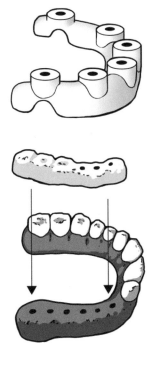

Types of surgical stents

Preparing for implant surgery is a major process for a dentist. It involves not only preparing the patient, but also the operatory and surgical staff for the procedure. Having taken preliminary impressions, the next step will involve sending the models to the dental laboratory for a diagnostic wax-up and surgical stent fabrication. Once the wax-up is approved and the surgical stent is ready, the next step would be to schedule the implant surgery and get prepared for the surgical therapy. For dentists that are just starting placement of dental implants, use of surgical stents are highly recommended.

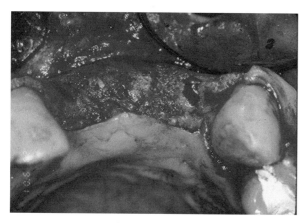

Dental implant placement
using surgical guide

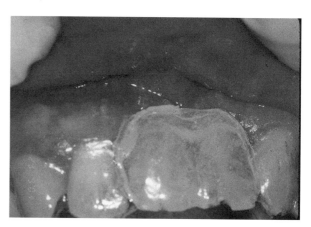

Nonlimiting stent in place

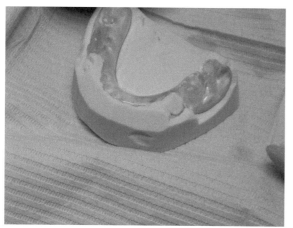

Posterior non limiting stent

Types of Surgical stents:

Surgical stents can be either fixed or variable. Variable position stents include those that are made with vacuumed formed acrylic and other materials over duplicate casts made from diagnostic wax-up. It takes into consideration the mesio-distal position of implant site as well as the width of the site.

Fixed stents do not allow for variation of the implant position from the one already planned. Most fixed stents utilize a 3D scan of the bone at the implant site, and help transmit this information to the optimal position in the mouth for implant placement. They usually are in the form of plastic, metal tubes and channels made in acrylic resins that determine the position of the dental implant prior to dental implant placement. [4]

More recently advanced techniques have been used for fabrication of surgical stents, and the design concepts for surgical stents can be classified further as non limiting stents, partially limiting stents and completely limiting stents.[3]

Nonlimiting stents provide the surgeon only with the ideal position of the implant restoration based on the diagnostic wax-up. It does not take into consideration angulation of the drill, therefore there is significant flexibility in the implant position. It also does not take into consideration site related factors such as presence of concavities in bone. Examples of non-limiting stents can include vacuum formed matrix with access holes that will place the dental implant in an optimal restorative position[3]

Partially limiting stents involve direction of the initial drill using a surgical guide and completing the rest of the surgery free hand. Fabrication of these stents involve to creation of a radiographic template which is converted to a surgical guide. The problem with these stents is that there is again a concern with ability to completely limit the angulation of drill. Most surgeries in the United States are performed using partially limiting stents due to cost effectiveness.[3]

Completely limiting stents create limits in angulation in the bucco-lingual and mesio-distal directions and control depths of burs by having stops on the drills. Two types exist, cast based stents and also CADCAM surgical guides.

The cast based technique combines analog technique done with bone sounding and periapical radiographs. The root is trans-positioned to the cast using imaging software, and a laboratory sleeve is converted in part with wires that produce a frame work around teeth. Polyvinylsiloxane is what forms the superstructure of the stent.

Fabricating CAD/CAM based surgical guides involve 4 steps:1) Fabrication of the template, 2) completion of CT Scan, 3) Implant planning using interactive software and 4) Fabrication of stereolithographic drill guide which will be used for surgery.[3]

CAD/CAM stents are considered to be the most accurate stents that currently exist. They promote use of flapless technique by allowing three dimensional visualization of the site so that adequate preoperative planning can be performed. They also allow pre-surgical master cast production so that provisional restorations can be created facilitating using of immediate dental implant placement and restoration but they are not completely without inaccuracy.

A study conducted on 61 placed dental implants using free hand technique with no surgical guide, tube, channel and Guided CAD/CAM stents found that while CAD/CAM stents had the least mesio-distal error, they were not as accurate as would have been desired in the bucco-lingual direction and tended to err towards implant placement to the palatal aspect.[5]

In evaluating the effect of surgical guides on dental implant surgery, it was found that most errors occurred in the position and angulation of the surgical guide, and that the surgeon's prior experience as well as the size of the site where the most important factors to creating errors that affected accuracy of dental implant placement using surgical guides.[5]

Advantages of Fixed Surgical Stents:

1) Simplicity. Better ease of implant placement.
2) Minimizes errors in angulation and positioning for dental implants.
3) More precision in the location of dental implants.
4) Allows visualization of potential restorative outcome during dental implant placement.
5) For anterior cases reduces risk of getting a poor esthetic result by direct guidance of implant position in comparison to adjacent teeth.
6) Allows avoidance of placement of implant into unfavorable positions such as in locations with concavities.
7) Accuracy. Especially for fixed positioned stents using 3D CT imaging, (completely limiting stents) they are able to prevent surprises during surgical therapy that would have resulted in changes in position of the dental implant to compensate for the bone changes. By showing the potential position of the dental implant restoration with regard to the existing bone in the site, unfavorable changes in bone density and bone width, and defects in bone can be identified and addressed prior to the surgical visit.

Required characteristics Surgical stents[8]:

1) Easy to place and remove from mouth.
2) It should be rigid and stable and stay in position during surgery drilling.
3) It should allow placement and removal of bite blocks if they are being used for the surgical procedure without obstruction.
4) It should not interfere with tissue reflection and also allow visualization of the surgical site where the surgery is being performed.

Restorative Temporization during implant integration:

Types of temporary restorations to utilize prior to permanent implant restorations include removable partial dentures, complete dentures, nesbite type removable restorations, Essix retainer type removable restorations, maryland bridges and also immediately loaded temporary restorations on dental implants. The type of permanent restoration to utilize is often determined in this early planning stage prior to dental implant placement to ensure optimal esthetic and functional outcomes.

For single tooth molar extractions, typically, most patients do not require provisionalization prior to dental implant placement because of the location in the mouth, but occasionally some highly esthetic conscious patients might want a temporary restoration fabricated to replace the missing posterior tooth while the implant is osseo-integrating. In such cases, nesbite type removable restoration that rest on adjacent teeth would be the best option available, although acrylic partials, retainer type devices and Maryland bridges are also viable options.

In the anterior areas of the mouth, the goal is to provide temporization which is both functional as well as esthetic. A number of factors are involved in treatment planning dental implants in the esthetic zone in the mouth. These factors include the location of the midline, the size of adjacent teeth, and the potential size of the implant restoration, the shade of adjacent teeth, the presence of excessive or deficient periodontal tissue as well as spacing or crowding of teeth. [1]

Temporization in the anterior zone is extremely important. Most patients will state a clear aversion to not having anterior temporary restorations even for a short period of time. Options for temporization of the partially edentulous anterior zone include removable acrylic partial dentures, Maryland bridges supported by adjacent teeth, Nesbyte type partials replacing single teeth, temporary restorations placed on the implants without occlusal loading on the dental implant, and permanent restoration of the dental implants with functional loading of the dental implant.

Keeping up with a need for esthetics in the maxillary anterior zone, the one stage technique with immediate restoration of dental implant with temporary or permanent restorations is done more frequently in this area of the mouth. The goal has been to provide patients with esthetic functional restorations while minimizing the wait time to receive their implant restorations. In the absence of significant bone loss requiring bone or soft tissue grafting, or replacement of endodontically and periodontally infected teeth, it is the recommended protocol in the esthetic zone, with success rate comparable or slightly higher than the two staged technique in the area.

Space analysis:

Consideration of available space is of paramount importance when planning dental implants for a number of reasons. 1.5mm to 2.5mm distance is the amount of space required between dental implants and adjacent teeth. This space allows the development of adequate contacts and contours around dental implant restorations as well as an adequate amount of soft tissue in between dental implants and adjacent teeth.[1]

To have adequate space to place a dental implant without any modification of dental implant protocol, a minimum space requirement involving a minimum of five to six millimeters (mm) in the bucco-lingual area and ten millimeters (mm) in the apical-coronal direction is needed for standard implant placement without any additional surgical intervention. The amount of space for requirements between implants and adjacent teeth should be a minimum of 1.5mm and 3mm between dental implants.[7] For ideal conditions, there should typically also be a minimum of eight millimeters of inter-occlusal space, this would allow an adequate amount of room for placement of abutments and dental implant crowns[7]. This would require 5mm for the abutment height, 3mm for soft tissue and for porcelain. [7] However options such as use of angled abutments and screw retained restorations are available when these ideal conditions do not exist.

In evaluating different areas of the mouth for implant placement, the space requirements for various teeth are varied. In premolar sites, an ideal amount of space in the mesio-distal direction ranging between six millimeters (mm) to nine millimeters would be required to allow placement of a 3.0mm to 4.0mm sized implant as well as maintain 1.5mm to 2.5mm between adjacent teeth and the dental implant. In the molar region the space requirement could vary between nine millimeters (mm) and twelve millimeters (mm) are within range to be adequate for a molar sized tooth. [1]

Single dental implant spaces that are more than 12mm in diameter could present esthetic problems resulting in oversized implant restorations. They might also require orthodontics to close the space further prior to dental implant restoration, or the use of two instead of one implant. As a result of the direct effect of space on the placement of dental implants, the recommendation is completion of orthodontic therapy, and restorations on adjacent teeth as well as other procedures that could affect the amount of space available for dental implant placement and restoration prior to actual dental implant placement.

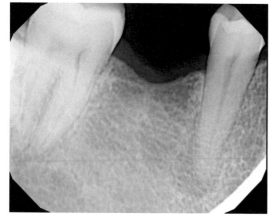

X-ray showing adequate molar space

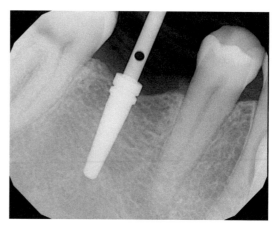

*X-ray showing adequate space
for molar implant*

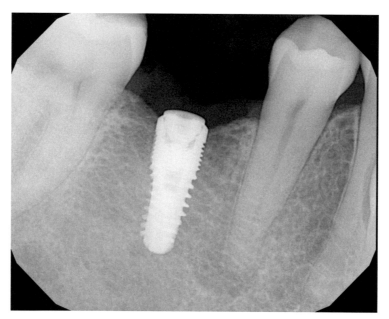

X-ray showing adequate space for molar restoration

When dental implants are placed too close to adjacent teeth, it can lead to loss of bone and soft tissue between the implants and adjacent teeth. Implants placed too far from adjacent teeth can lead to cantilever forces on the implant restoration. [3] It can also lead to implant restorations with open contacts, or excessively large non esthetic restorations. When inadequate space exists, it can be corrected with full coverage restorations on adjacent teeth if only minor spatial disparities exist and adjacent require restorations or Orthodontics. Second molar in x-ray requires molar up-righting prior to dental implant restoration.

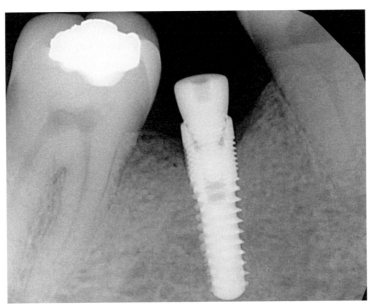

X-ray showing inadequate space for molar sized implant crown

During evaluation of inter-occlusal space, in order to adequately allow for placement of implant restorations that are esthetic and functional, an inter-occlusal space of about 8mm is needed for straight abutments. [7] If the inter-occlusal space is less than 8mm, a complex situation is created requiring the use of angled abutments or a more facial location of the dental implants.

Typically, the use of a diagnostic wax up would allow visualization of the potential restorative outcome prior to fabrication of surgical stent and implant placement. Excessive inter-occlusal space might necessitate use of pink porcelain to compensate for lost periodontal tissue or result in longer restorations in comparison to adjacent teeth. It is therefore crucial to evaluate inter-occlusal space prior to treatment planning dental implants so that should secondary procedures such as bone grafting be needed, they can be performed prior to dental implant placement.

Chapter 1 Summary: Sequence of Dental Implant therapy:

1) Completion of Clinical exams and Initial radiographs
2) Diagnostic casts, wax up, evaluation for provisional restorations and completion of specialized radiographs (CT scans) if needed.
3) Discussion of treatment options and decision of what type of permanent restoration will be utilized.
4) Completion of any necessary dental treatment including extraction of hopeless teeth, periodontal treatment, endodontic therapy, restorative treatment and new restorations in adjacent teeth, prior to dental implant surgery.
5) Construction of provisional restorations during dental implant osteointegration for submerged technique.
6) Construction of the surgical stent.
7) Fabrication of provisional restorations if non submerged technique is being utilized
8) Surgical Implant placement.
9) Osteo-integration followed by second stage surgery if needed.
10) Prosthetic phase.

CHAPTER 2

Assessment of conditions that can affect dental implant placement

As part of initial examination, teeth are screened for the presence of potentially damaging conditions such as periodontal disease and dental caries, the presence of fractured teeth or restorations, discolorations, and infections and these conditions addressed prior to dental implant placement. Periodontitis, peri-apical infections and caries should be addressed prior to starting dental implant placement in order to prevent the success of dental implant placement from being impacted due to dental disease.

Typically, when tooth loss occurs due to periodontal disease, a significant amount of bone loss can occur around the tooth. So especially in the esthetic zone, extraction and bone grafting prior to placement of the dental implant is the course of action in order to prevent esthetic complications that can occur due to having a restoration located more apically than adjacent teeth.

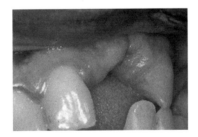

Picture showing site with bone and soft tissue loss due to gum disease that
will require significant grafting prior to dental implant placement

Some studies have found a detrimental effect of placing dental implants immediately into sites with prior infections such as increased incidence of peri-implantitis. To err on the side of caution, using a delayed approach involving extraction and bone grafting prior to implant placement is recommended especially if just recently placing dental implants.

With regard to periodontitis, endodontic lesions or dental caries in adjacent teeth, it has been recommended that the dental disease should be addressed prior to placing the dental implant. In the case of periodontal disease, this would prevent re-infection of the implant site by adjacent micro-flora from other teeth with periodontal disease. Endodontic lesions adjacent to dental implant sites can also detrimentally affect the success of dental implants by damaging the viability of bone cells in the area.

During the initial dental implant assessment, the goal is to assess the condition of adjacent teeth and screen for dental diseases and other pre-existing conditions. Certain relative contraindications can exist for dental implant placement. These are comprised of local and medical factors. Medical contraindications for dental implant placement can include acute infection, severe bronchitis, emphysema, severe anemia, uncontrolled diabetes and hypertension, abnormal liver function, psychological illness involving neurological disorders like autism and down syndrome as well as psychiatric disorders such as schizophrenia.[9]

While most patients that are having dental implants will be in the Academy of Anesthesiology (ASA) classification of P1 or P2, which means that they are either healthy, or that they have a mild systemic condition that is usually controlled. For significantly medically compromised patients, a medical clearance is required and typically the implant procedure is delayed until their systemic condition is more controlled.

Local factors that can affect implant placement include proximity to vital structures, acute infection, inadequate bone width, height or length, soft tissue and jaw pathology, TM joint disease, salivary gland pathology, maxillary sinus pathology, uncontrolled periodontal disease, Trigeminal neuralgia, orofacial dysthesia and orofacial dyskinesia.[11].

Anatomy affecting dental implant placement:

In performing dental implant surgery in the mouth, a number of anatomic considerations need to be addressed during treatment planning. Anatomic structures such as the maxillary sinus in the posterior maxilla, the nasopalatine nerve in the anterior maxilla, and the inferior alveolar nerve, mental foramen and nerve, and genial tubercles in the mandible have to be identified radiographically and clinically, prior to dental implant treatment planning and selection of dental implants.

The size and the location of the maxillary sinus can affect the amount of available bone height to place dental implants into. The roots of the first and second maxillary molars are in direct contact with the maxillary sinus floor. Assessment of the bone level at the posterior maxilla, as well as bone quality can be done utilizing CT scans. To compensate for a pneumatized sinus, use of shorter dental implants, or planning a sinus lift prior to dental implant placement or simultaneously with placement is often necessary. Sinus elevation will be reviewed later in the book.

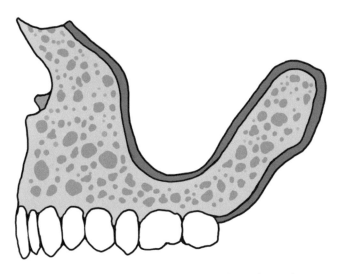

Sinus limitations that can affect dental implant placement

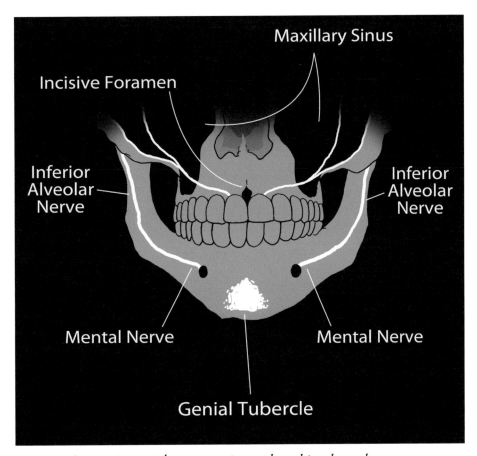

Anatomic considerations prior to dental implant placement

The naso palatine foramen and nerve fibers are located posteriorly between the two central incisors. Their location should be identified and taken into consideration when treatment planning anterior implants. Typically, there are not many complications that can occur if it is impinged on, but the recommendation is to have a more facial flap to avoid affecting the nerve bundle in addition to avoiding dental placement into the nerve bundle. In rare instances when it is impinged on, tingling sensation from numbness in tissue in the palate could occur.[13]

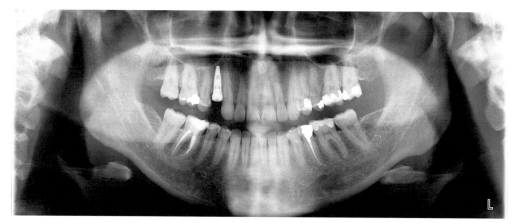
Panorex showing implant placement without impinging on maxillary sinus

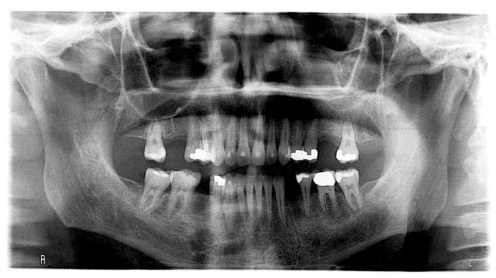
Panorex showing reduced maxillary ridge height due to pneumatized sinus

In the mandible, the mandibular nerve, the third branch of the Trigeminal nerves gives rise to the inferior alveolar nerve after it exits the mandibular canal. The location of the inferior alveolar nerve is crucial when determining the length of implants to place. Damage to the inferior alveolar nerve can result in damage that can be transcient or permanent, and manifest as paresthesia, dysthesia, analgesia or anesthesia(complete loss of sensation).[12] It is therefore essential to correctly identify it on radiographs prior to dental implant placement, if unable to identify on panoramic and peri-apical x-rays, a CT scan is necessary to clearly identify it.

The Inferior alveolar nerve divides into the mental nerve and the incisive nerve branches at the premolar area.[14] Anterior to the mental foramen are the branches of the incisive nerve that extend as far forward as the lateral incisors.[13] Damage to the inferior alveolar nerve can result in numbness in the lower lip, mucosa and the chin in the area. Studies have shown that implants should be placed at least 2mm or more above the location of the nerve. Since the location of the nerve might sometimes not be readily visualized on conventional radiographs, use of CT scan to locate the mandibular canal is often implemented when implants are planned in the premolar and molar region to prevent nerve impingment.[10]

During dental implant placement in the posterior mandible, when there is impingement of the mandibular canal, the goal is to take a CT scan as soon as possible and remove the implant if the inferior alveolar nerve is affected. Juodzbalys and colleagues described steps for addressing Inferior Alveolar nerve injuries:[59]

1) Stage 1. **Recording general risk factors** in the mandible. Patients are required to sign informed consent forms as well as undergo a neurosensory exam before dental implant placement to ensure that there was no nerve damage prior to dental implant placement and the patient's gender is noted because females and older adults are more prone to neurosensory deficits.

2) Stage II: **Involves the record of intraoperative risk factors.** Pain or sensation that feels like an electrical shock sensation that can occur during anesthesia administration or bone preparation is not indicative of permanent nerve injury and can occur after contact with even a small needle.

3) Stage III: **Contact with patient after Anesthesia wears off.** Dentists should record patient complaint related to altered sensation and perform a neurosensory exam documenting the results after surgery but no later than 36 hours after the anesthesia wears off. If patient has sensory complaints related to nerve injury, they are assigned to the inferior alveolar nerve injury group.

4) Stage IV: **Post op examination, risk factor evaluation and diagnosis statement.** Starts with a neurosensory exam to evaluate sensory lesion, neurosensory mapping of areas affected and pictures if needed. CT Scan x-rays are then recommended to assess radiographically for if the nerve injury is caused by dental implant placement. Completion of diagnosis statement based on patient complaints, Inferior alveolar nerve neurosensory exam results and radiographic assessment. Patient should be referred to appropriate specialist for further assessment.

5) Stage V: **Treatment of Numbness. Psychological treatment** involving immediate information, explanation and support for patient.

Physiologic treatment involving implant removal if it is in any way proximal to or contacting the mandibular canal, or patient has signs of damage to Inferior alveolar nerve. Following removal cleaning of debris or irritant that is close to the nerve is performed. Placement of bone graft is not recommended at this time because it can affect nerve recovery.

Medications to treat altered sensation or numbness of Inferior Alveolar nerve can include 3 week course with steroids and NSAIDs. Steroid therapy can include Dexamethasone 4mg, with 2 tabs every morning for 3 days and 1 tablet of Oral Prednisone every morning for the preceding 3 days. Also, IV steroids involving 1ml of Dexamethasone 4mg/ml can also be used for treating IAN injury.

Continued use of Ice packs over the first 24 hours and intermittently for the first 1 week can also be helpful in treating nerve injury and helping to prevent permanent nerve damage.

Additional medication and therapy such as use of antidepressants and transcutaneous nerve stimulation can also be recommended.

6) Stage VI: **1 week post-op examination (Neurosensory and clinical exams).** The exam is used to monitor recovery of Inferior alveolar nerve after injury. Mapping of neurosensory deficit and comparison to previous exams and comparison pictures can also be taken of the site. If there is

paresthesia, the recommendation is exams every week for the first 3 weeks and every 2-3 weeks for the 12 weeks after.

7) Stage VII: **1 week post-op treatment.** Psychological support for patient is continued. Medications are recommended including continued use of 800mg Motrin three times daily for 3 weeks. If necessary additional use of Motrin 800mg three times daily for an additional 3 weeks can be implemented. For micro-neurosurgical care, if dysesthesia or complete anesthesia is present, the patient should be referred to a Neurosurgeon. Additional treatments can continue including use of drugs such antidepressants and additional physiologic therapy.

8) Stage VII: **12 weeks postoperative examination.** Appointment is used to continue to monitor Inferior alveolar nerve sensory function recovery and neurosensory deficit mapping and additional photographs are taken of the affected areas.

9) Stage VIII: **12 weeks postoperative treatment.** Continued medications if needed. If no signs of sensory function recovery is noted then patient should have micro-neurosurgical treatment to try to help repair the nerve damage.

Chapter 2 Summary: Factors that affect Dental implant placement

1) Medical and anatomic conditions exist that impact dental implant placement.

2) Medical contraindications to dental implant placement can exist for patients who have acute infection, severe bronchitis, emphysema, uncontrolled diabetes and hypertension, patients with neurologic disorders such as down syndrome and autism as well as psychiatric disorders like schizophrenia and Patients on prolonged use of medications like Fusomax.

3) The naso palatine foramen, mental nerve, inferior alveolar nerve, maxillary sinus and genial tubercle are anatomic structures that should be identified during dental implant treatment planning.

4) A CT Scan should be performed if dental implant placement is planned in the posterior maxilla and mandible due to the presence of the inferior alveolar nerve or potential for pneumatization of the maxillary sinus.

5) When the sinus is pneumatized, sinus augmentation or use of shorter dental implants should be implemented.

6) Typically, a minimum height of 2mm should be present between the location of dental implant and the nerve to prevent nerve damage.

7) Damage to the nasopalatine nerve can result in a tingling numbness palatal to the maxillary incisors.

8) Damage to the inferior alveolar nerve can result in damage to the lower lip, mucosa and chin on the affected side.

CHAPTER 3

Dental Implant Components and Protocols for Dental Implant surgery

A number of components are utilized during dental implant placement and restoration. During surgical therapy, the components include the dental implant itself, a cover screw and healing abutment that is utilized to protect the internal connection of the dental implant when utilizing a two staged dental implant placement protocol. Platform mounts attached directly to dental implants might be used during surgery in order to better approximate angulation of dental implants in relation to other teeth in the mouth. These mounts are either removed at the end of the surgery or retained for a one staged dental implant placement.

Healing abutments are components that are utilized to adapt tissue around an implant in anticipation of a permanent abutment and dental implant restoration. Healing abutments are placed following osteo-integration during a two staged or submerged dental implant placement protocol. It usually replaces a cover screw, and helps to adapt tissue around dental implants in preparation for permanent abutments and dental implant restorations.

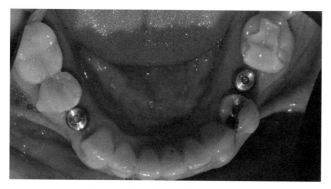
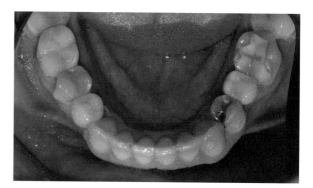

Premolar dental implants   *Premolar restoration*

Dental implant components include the dental implant itself which comes with either a cover screw, healing abutment, permanent abutment or temporary abutment. One staged dental implants include the dental implant with the abutments or platform mount attached already. More recently, the attached abutments are also detachable, and they can be converted to a two staged protocol by using a cover screw instead of the attached abutment.

Restorative components for replacing partially or fully edentulous sites with fixed restorations include: Impression copings, analogs, standard machined abutments, UCLA abutments, zirconia abutments, angled abutments, uni-abutments, torque wrenches, and abutment drivers. If one stage technique is being utilized, the dental implant already has an abutment attached to the implant at time of placement.

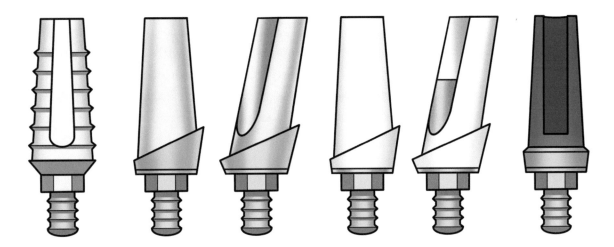

Types of abutments

The one staged protocol was developed by ITI dental implant company in Switzerland and involves the fixture extending through soft tissue during dental implant placement.[1] It requires only one surgery allowing the fixture and abutment to be placed. It also allows not only healing of the bone around the implant during the osteo-integration process, but also the formation and maturation of soft tissue around the abutment. During treatment planning this technique is performed either with a flapless technique usually utilizing CT guided technology or with of a muco-periosteal flap utilizing either a guided or non-guided protocol.

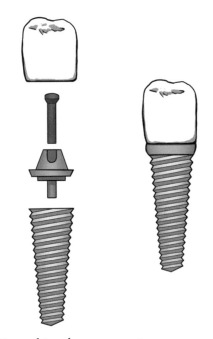

Dental implant restorative components

The two staged technique involves placement of dental implants in a submerged position utilizing a cover screw, and then placement of an abutment as a second stage following osteo-integration of the dental implant. It was originally described by Brannemark in 1969. A major advantage of utilizing the two stage technique is that any additional soft tissue and bone augmentation can be able to be completed prior to final dental implant restoration. [1]

In reviewing success rate of both procedures, Balshi TJ et al performed a retrospective study to evaluate single stage free hand protocol involving one stage implant placement without CT guided technology, one stage implant placement utilizing guided technology with CT Scan generated surgical guides, and two stage submerged technique utilizing cover screws at time of dental implant placement and second stage surgery after implant healing. They found 10% higher success rate for one staged versus two staged dental implant placement.[15]

Their study found that the single staged technique resulted in statistically significantly higher success than the two staged technique, regardless of whether it involved use of guided or non-guided techniques. Both single stage techniques did not have statistical difference in success rate. The possible advantages they felt were provided by the single stage technique included the ability of patients to receive fixed restorations on the same day allowing esthetics and function during healing phase as well as that the provisional restoration can protect the sutured mucosal tissue against masticatory forces or trauma.[15] Single staged dental implant placement can utilize non-guided protocol without use of CT scan technology, or it can be performed with a CT guided technique with the goal of improving accuracy and precision.

Indications for Guided Technology:

CT guided technology for dental implant placement can be utilized with either a flapless technique or with a muco-periosteal flap. The goal is to improve accuracy and precision of dental implant placement by working backwards utilizing possible restorative outcomes, and relating them to the anatomic factors affecting the implant site. CT scans allow characteristics of bone in the implant site to be viewed in three dimensions allowing for more accurate planning. [16] According to Orentlicher et al the indications for CT guided technology include [16,17]:

1) When planning for three or more dental implants.
2) Proximity to vital anatomy.
3) Proximity to Adjacent teeth.
4) Questionable bone volume.
5) Implant position that is critical to restoration.
6) Flapless placement of dental implant is planned.
7) For medically involved patients that require minimal chair time.
8) For areas with alterations in bone anatomy such as bone with prior trauma.
9) Fully edentulous cases.

While guided technology presents with advantages such as increased precision and accuracy, it is restorative driven so it allows the end result to be first visualized, as the implant crown and then ensures placement of the implant into the right position. [17] When flapless technique is being utilized even for single dental implant placement, use of a CT scan is highly recommended.

Other advantages of Guided technology include reduced time from dental implant placement to loading, less surgical trauma for patients as well as decreased post operative sequelae such as pain and swelling, and an overall shorter recovery time because not as much tissue access is needed for surgical visualization due to the earlier planning with the CT scan and surgical guide.[17]

Dental Implant placement using Mucoperiosteal Flap and Flapless Technique:

Routinely, full thickness mucoperiosteal flaps have been utilized for dental implant surgery especially in areas of the mouth that are proximal to vital structures or might have bone concavities present, or present with possible concerns about the bone quantity. The advantage of mucoperiosteal flaps has been the ability to have adequate visualization and access of the surgical site. Potential concerns with muco-periosteal flap are due to their increased risk of post-operative discomfort following dental implant surgery. While the mucoperiosteal flap is still regarded as the standard of care, with increased technological advances present such as CT guided scans and surgical guides, more surgeons are increasing use of flapless technique which can present with less surgical trauma.

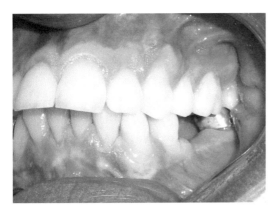

Dental implant used for molar replacement

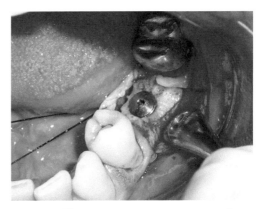

Papilla preserving mucoperiosteal flap for implant placement

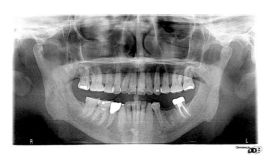

X-ray for molar replacement

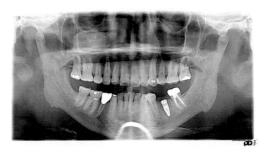

X-ray of molar implant

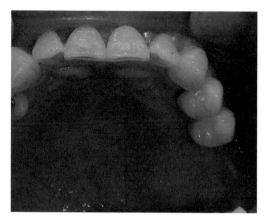
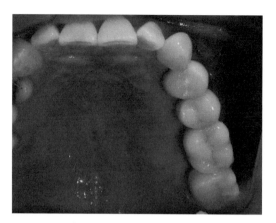

Patient missing two maxillary molars

Replacement of missing molars with maxillary dental implants

A number of requirements exist for selection of patients that are having dental implants utilizing the flapless technique. These include adequate amounts of attached gingiva and bone volume and density as well as a width of 5mm or more of bone being present in the site receiving the implant where no additional bone augmentation is being performed. [18]

Sites that have less than 5mm of bone require additional surgical procedures including split crest technique or bone augmentation and these techniques have to be completed prior to dental implant placement. Block grafting or bone augmentation using particulate bone grafts and collagen barriers are needed prior to dental implant placement because the bone present is not adequate.

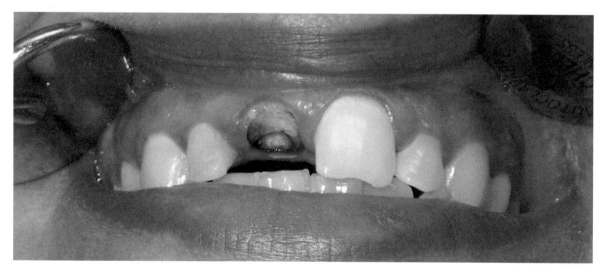

Immediate placement with flapless technique

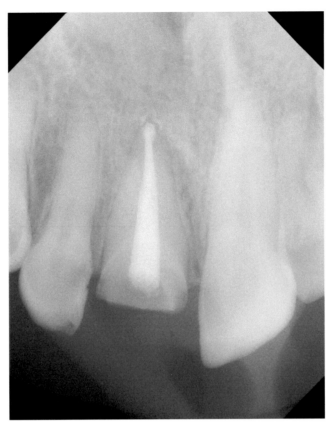

X-ray

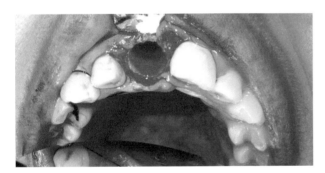

Atraumatic extraction

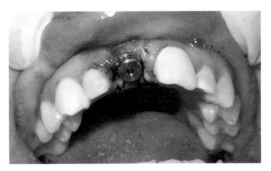

Healing abutment placed

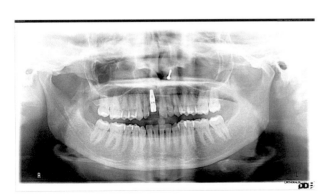

X-ray of implant placement

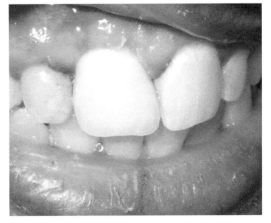

Dental implant restored

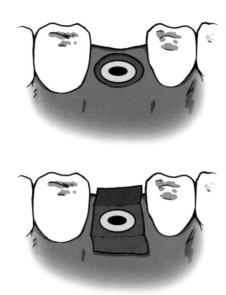

Flapless versus muco-periosteal flap technique

Advantages of flapless technique compared to muco-periosteal flaps involve decreased discomfort for patients as well as less recession and tissue shrinkage during healing. Less tissue trauma also results from the technique as well as faster post-operative healing.[18]

The disadvantage of the flapless technique is that it requires careful pre-operative planning and is very technique sensitive. Ability to sound and determine quality of the underlying bone using sounding techniques and CT scans are paramount to the success of the surgery in addition to choosing the appropriate dental implant size. In addition, because the surgical site is not clearly visualized, care has to be taken to prevent perforation of bone and also to make sure that vital anatomic structures are not impinged on.

Use of dental implants that are wider than needed for the ostectomy can lead to buccal, or lingual bone resorption over time resulting in fenestration and dehiscence defects. Using standard implant size corresponding to bone width are recommended to prevent loss of bone and preserve the cortical plate.

The goal of the flapless technique is to preserve bone and tissue in the implant site. Surgical access can be achieved with a scalpel or with a tissue punch biopsy. During dental implant placement, CT scans are completed first, and then sent with impressions to dental laboratories and companies that use CADCAM technology to complete fabrication of surgical guide. Because even the slightest deviation in dental implant placement can be able to impair the restorative outcome, use of a surgical guide is of paramount importance when utilizing the flapless technique. These guides are made prior to the surgery and guide in the positioning and placement of dental implants. Due to the precision of fixed limiting surgical guides, they allow the placement of the implants in positions that take into consideration anatomy of the implant site as well as the best position for esthetics.

Chapter 3 Summary: Implant Surgical Protocols

1) Protocols for Dental Implant surgery involve a two staged protocol with implant submerged during healing, and a one staged protocol that involves use of provisional or permanent dental implant restorations at time of dental implant placement.

2) Some of the advantages of the one stage protocol for dental implant placement is that it allows for the maturation of bone and soft tissue when temporaries are used prior to permanent restoration. The provisional restoration protects the surgical site immediately after surgery, less trauma to sutures and operated tissue occurs as well as less wait time for patients to have functional restorations.

3) Advantages of the two staged protocol is that it can be utilized for implants that might not have stability to support a restoration at time of placement. It can offer the advantage of non-disturbed implant healing during the osteointegration process which is especially important for sites with simultaneous dental implant placement and grafts. As well as it is advantageous in sites where due to esthetic, anatomic or functional reasons, immediate loading may negatively affect implant healing in the site.

4) CT guided technology has been vital in increasing precision during dental implant placement. By allowing pre surgical viewing of the implant site so that pre surgical planning including ideal positions for implant placement and restoration, and fabrication of surgical guides can be completed.

5) CT Scan technology has been used for the fabrication of surgical stents that are fixed stents, these stent can be fabricated using CAD /CAM technology, this allows for fabrication of a master model prior to the surgery as well as a stereolithographic stent which restricts the angulation and depth of the implant drills to ensure that there is not a deviation from the optimal site for placement determined from the CT scan.

6) Use of CT guided technology has also increased precision for flapless technique allowing surgery to be placed more accurately by providing information about the anatomic site.

7) CT guided technology has also improved proficiency with the one stage technique allowing for the fabrication of provisional and permanent dental implant restorations that are more accurately fabricated prior to the implant surgery based on specifications from the CT Scan. They allow patients to have access to esthetic functional restorations sooner rather later by having a master model prior to dental implant placement.

CHAPTER 4

Late, Early and Immediate implant placement

When treatment planning teeth replacement with dental implants, one of the key factors to consider is whether to place the dental implant during time of extraction (immediate placement) or to extract the tooth and place the dental implant after a period of time to allow bone healing prior to dental implant placement (delayed placement). Both protocols present with advantages and disadvantages.

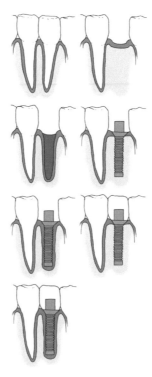

Immediate versus Delayed dental Implant Placement

Delayed dental implant placement involves placement of dental implants after allowing a period of time after extraction for bone healing to occur. This is the favored technique for teeth that present with trauma, endodontic or periodontal infection or extensive soft or hard tissue defects. It is also the favored technique when the tooth to be extracted presents with a thin tissue biotype. The healing time prior to dental implant placement allows improvements to occur in the site, as a result of bone grafting and soft tissue grafting prior to dental implant placement so that problems caused by thin biotype of tissue can be able to be addressed. In cases of delay placement and restoration, the implant is not loaded immediately after surgery, allowing the implant to heal undisturbed until osteointegration is completed.

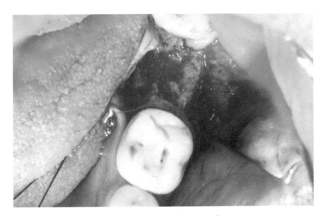
Delayed dental implant placement

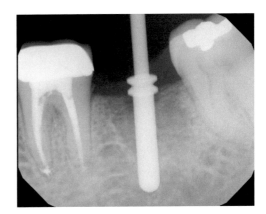
Delayed dental implant placement

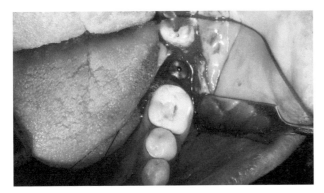
Dental implant placed

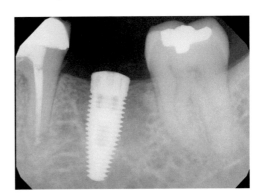
X-ray of delayed implant placement

Immediate dental implant placement offers the advantage of having a shorter amount of time for implant integration by eliminating the amount of wait time necessary for healing of the bone to occur prior to dental implant placement. It also allows the position of the dental implant to replicate the prior tooth position in the dental arch that it is replacing. The bone cells that are also available after the extraction are able to provide a benefit during osteointegration by having viable cells readily available in the extraction socket.

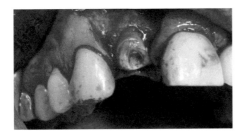

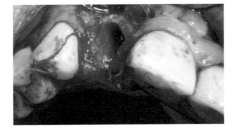

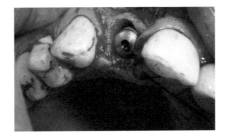

Immediate dental implant placement with bone graft in place

Root Fractures involve fractures of the root affecting cementum, dental and pulp.[62] Root fractures can be horizontal or vertical in nature. Horizontal fractures are the most common types of root fractures with most fractures predominantly in the anterior maxilla area specifically around central incisors.62 Most horizontal fractures occur in the middle third of roots, but less frequently in the apical and coronal one-third of roots.

The most common etiology of fractures can involve physical trauma such as from falls, automobile accidents and sporting events.[63] Other causes can include excessive occlusal trauma and occlusal overload. Treatment for occlusal trauma can include repositioning and splinting of the fractured segment, performing root canals and restoring the fractured tooth or Extraction.63 When extraction is treatment planned, immediate implant placement is typically the treatment of choice when the alveolus is intact.

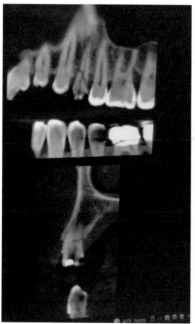 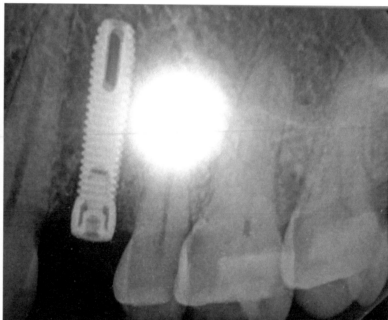

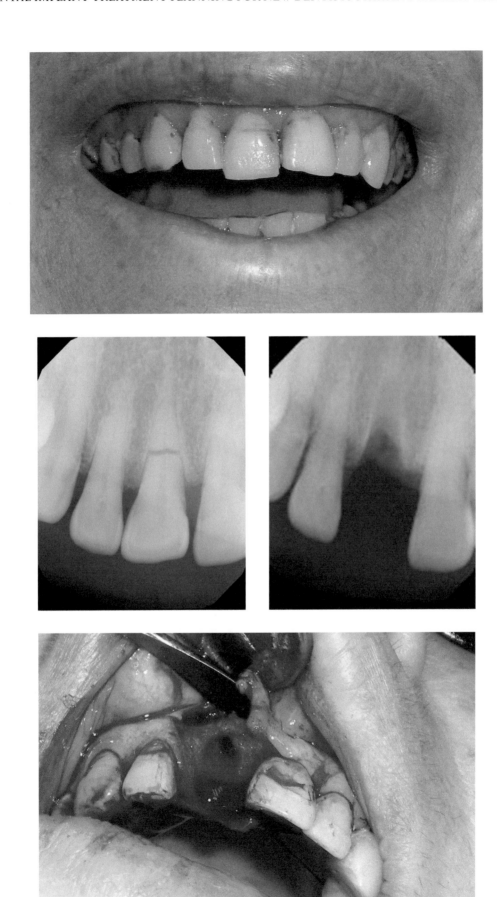

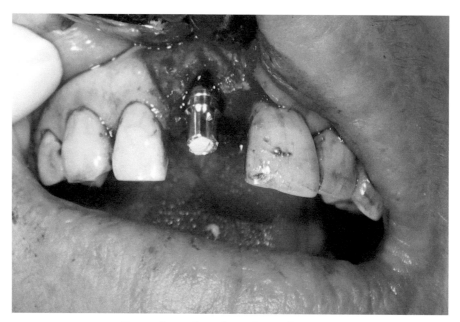

Immediate dental implant placement

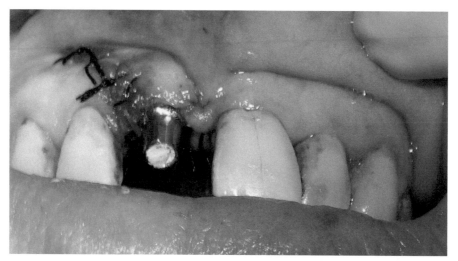

Immediate dental implant placement

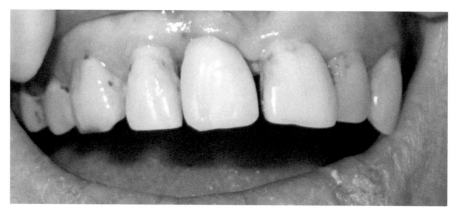

Immediate placement and restoration with temporary crown

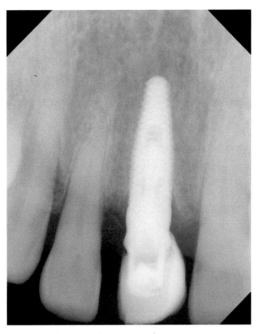

X-ray of immediate temporary restoration

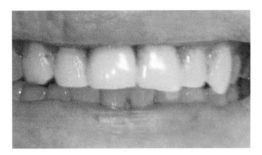

Final restoration in place

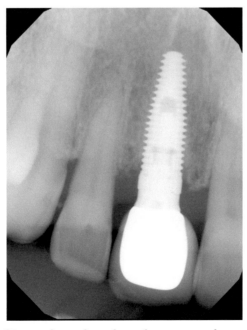

X-ray of Immediate dental implant restored permanently

A number of criteria have to be met for the immediate dental implant protocol to be utilized. One of these is the extraction socket characteristics. The closer to being intact that a socket is, the less chances of needing bone grafting and other socket preservation techniques. Salama's classification system for extraction sockets was created based on defect morphology of the extraction socket as well as the regenerative potential which is based on the number of walls present in an extraction socket. While a four walled socket is regarded as an intact socket not requiring any regeneration technique, the socket with three or less walls implies a need for regeneration procedure. The goal of classification is to identify socket defects prior to extraction to correct the socket architecture. [19]

Salama Type 1 classification refers to an intact socket containing four walls. There is adequate bone available, and apico-coronally, the bone crest that will contain the neck of the implant is in close proximity to the CEJ of adjacent teeth and the buccal bone is also adequate. This classification is usually ideal for immediate dental implant placement. [19]

Salama Type 2 classification refers to an extraction socket which requires grafting due to moderately comprised extraction site that needs regeneration. It may include sites with dehiscence greater than 5mm, the extraction socket might have discrepancy between osseous crest and CEJ of adjacent teeth as well as significant facial recession. They advocate the use of extrusion prior to extraction to attempt to improve the architecture of the socket and improve the bone volume of the socket available to engage a dental implant as a means of correcting the reduced regenerative potential found in type 2 sockets. [19]

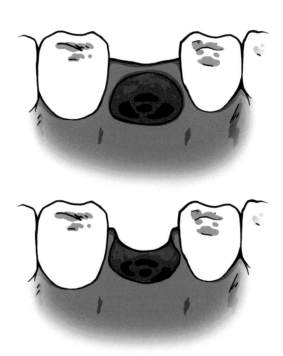

4 walled versus 3 walled extraction sockets

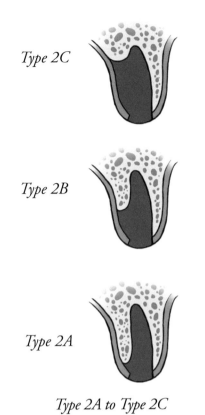

Type 2C

Type 2B

Type 2A

Type 2A to Type 2C
Chu Dehiscence Sub-Classifications

Salama type 3 classification refers to bone loss in an apical direction as well as buccal that is in need of extensive bone and soft tissue grafting it also refers to socket sites with severe loss of facial plate as well as those with circumferential and angular defects. To address sockets with these severe defects, a two stepped approach is recommended involving bone grafting and regenerative procedures prior to dental implant placement. [19]

Chu et al reclassified current classification of dehiscence defects with three classes[58] ranging from 1 to 3, and subdivided their class 2 classification into divided into additional sub-classifications. According to their classification system, type one involves labial bone plate that is intact with soft tissue that is also intact. Their type two involves sites with adequate soft tissue with osseous defects that indicate partial or complete loss of labial bone.

Type 2A refers to coronal one third loss of buccal plate (5-6mm from the gingival margin) and soft tissue that is still intact. Type 2B involves absence of coronal two third of the buccal plate (7-9mm from free gingival margin) and Type 2C involves absence of the apical one third of the buccal plate (more than 10mm from gingival margin). Type 3 dehiscence classification according to Chu et al involves midfacial recession presenting loss of labial bone and also loss of soft tissue.[20] As the level of dehiscence of the buccal plate increases, the potential for immediate implant placement reduces. While they recommend that immediate placement can be performed for type 1 and most type 2 defects, type 3 defects require a delayed dental implant placement approach. [20]

Other classifications systems have been used for classifying extraction sockets. According to Greenstein et al in classifying extraction sockets, extraction sockets can be classified into four categories. In categorizing the socket characteristics with type of protocol and therapy needed, they indicated that while only type 1 and type 2 extraction site types are ideal for immediate dental implant placement and require minimal bone grafting, type 3 and 4 require extensive bone and soft tissue grafting and therefore should be treated using a delayed dental implant placement protocol rather than an immediate protocol. Poor dental implant stability could occur if bone grafting is not completed first in type 3 and 4 cases. [21]

Recently, the ITI Consensus conference in 2008 changed from earlier terms that classified implant placement protocols as Immediate, delayed immediate and delayed protocols instead to Immediate, Early and Late placement protocols:[60,61]

1) **Immediate implant placement:** Placement of dental implant at time of tooth extraction.
2) **Early Placement with soft tissue healing:** occurs at 4-8 weeks after teeth extraction. Involves significant soft tissue healing and slight bone healing.

3) **Early implant placement with partial bone healing:** occurs at 12-16 weeks after tooth extraction. Involves complete soft tissue healing and partial bone healing.

4) **Late implant placement:** occurs after 6 months after tooth extraction. Complete bone and soft tissue healing occurs after tooth extraction prior to dental implant placement.

Chapter Summary 4: Delayed and Immediate Dental Implant placement

1) Late implant placement involves implant placement after 6months, while Early placement occurs from 4-16 weeks after extraction.

2) Immediate dental implant placement involves dental implant placement at time of teeth extraction.

3) Delayed implant placement is advocated for sites that will require further site development prior to dental implant placement such as sites that require augmentation of underlying bone, sites with apical defects, teeth with prior endodontic and periodontal infections, as well as healthy sites that have thin biotypes.

4) Areas in the esthetic zone that present with high esthetic risks such as areas with high smile lines and areas that require papilla preservation techniques might be sites that would benefit from additional site development and will benefit from delayed implant plant placement.

5) Sites that present with adequate tissue support and require minimal bone and soft tissue augmentation will benefit from immediate implant placement.

6) Salama and Salama classification system classified bone quality in extraction sockets, and noted that their class1 category dealt with extractions sites with good bone regenerative potential that do not need bone grafting, and less than 5mm of bone loss expected. Category 2 deal with sites with potential of more that 5mm dehiscence present that might need extrusion prior to extraction and category 3 which had most of the root contained in a defect and would require extensive bone grafting prior to dental implant placement.

7) Areas in the anterior zone that present with an adequate bone support and thick gingival biotypes are also good candidates for immediate dental implant placement.

8) Immediate dental implant placement offers that advantage of shorter wait times for dental implant restoration, ability to duplicate the prior tooth position with the implant placement, ability to maintain soft tissue contours and preserve interdental papilla.

9) Delayed dental implant placement allows the ability to improve bone and soft tissue support prior to dental implant placement.

CHAPTER 5

Site preparation prior and during Dental Implant placement.

Dental implant placement is now primarily restoration driven. The goal is to have optimal site locations that are also are ideal sites appropriate for restorations. Consistent with restoration driven implant placement, when dental implants sites are deficient in width, height, or length, or when soft tissue deficiencies are present, it is recommended that the defect correction occur prior to dental implant placement.

Use of bone grafting prior to dental implant placement is recommended when less than 5mm of bone diameter is present. The bone graft performed can either be an autogenous graft, particulate or block allograft, or an alloplast utilizing synthetic bone. Bone grafting can be performed in combination with collagen membranes to enhance the result of augmentation. The goal is to have adequate bone for implant placement and then place dental implants when there is adequate bone to support a dental implant.

According to Kazor el, the prerequisites for optimal dental implant placement include adequate bone volume (sufficient amount of bone in the horizontal, vertical and contour of the bone), as well as optimal dental implant position, mesial, distal, apico-coronal, buccolingual and angulation for dental implant placement. Both conditions are needed for healthy tissue around dental implants, and ideal emergence profile.[22]

A number of classification systems have been developed to classify both bone quality, quantity and overall contour of bone. The classification system by Lekholm and Zarb is based on the residual edentulous ridge remaining following extractions, and is based on a 5 point scale ranging from A-E, with Category A representing a still intact ridge with no basal bone absorption and E representing a severely deficient edentulous ridge. [23]

The Misch and Judy Classification of bone classifies bone into a range from adequate to deficient. The four divisions range from A-D, where A represents adequate bone with more than 5mm width that does not require any augmentation. According to the classification, B represents barely sufficient ridge width of 2.5-5mm width and requires additional bone or soft tissue augmentation, and C refers to compromised bone that requires osteoplasty and soft and hard tissue augmentation. D refers to deficient bone requiring substantial bone augmentation. [24]

During the treatment planning phase for dental implants, a number of additional procedures can be planned early such as bone grafts and soft tissue grafts to increase tissue around implant site in order to maximize chances for a successful outcome. Procedures such as socket preservation performed at time of tooth extractions are also necessary in preparing dental implant sites to receive dental implants.

For areas with thin soft tissue biotype or where defects in soft tissue exist, or sites with minimal attached tissue present, use of soft tissue grafts are recommended. The use of soft tissue grafts such as free gingival or connective tissue graft and pedicle grafts can increase keratinized tissue, resulting in adequate support around dental implants and restorations.

Optimal dental implant position involves location of implant in the edentulous space that is optimal in three dimensions, mesio-distal, bucco-lingual and apico-coronal as it relates to the implant restoration[22].

When looking at the mesio-distal dental implant position, a minimum of 2mm distance is recommended to exist between the dental implant and adjacent teeth. This is to ensure that there is adequate osteointegration and also reduced risk of damage to adjacent teeth. The recommendation was made to take into consideration the width of the PDL. It is also being recommended that the distance cervically should be 2mm between implant face and natural tooth, and 3mm between adjacent implants to account for the interproximal tooth contact as well interdental papilla area. The maintaining of these space requirements has been shown to reduce bone loss inter-proximally and support the interproximal papilla form. [22]

In the bucco-lingual dimension positioning of dental implants, a recommendation of 2-4mm of space is recommended between the implant collar and the longitudinal axis and cervical contours to allow adequate cervical contouring of the restoration. A recommendation was made for a minimum amount of bone of 1.8mm on the facial aspect of dental implants to be able to maintain implant tissue health, and prevent facial positioning as well as dehiscence of the facial bone around the dental implant. [22]

When positioning the dental implant in the apico-coronal dimension, a number of factors have to be considered such as the overall bone morphology, implant diameter and the presence or absence of recession. The dental implant collar should be 2mm apical to the cemento-enamel junction (CEJ) of adjacent teeth if there is no recession present, and 3mm from the CEJ of adjacent teeth when recession exists around adjacent teeth. [22]

Implants that are positioned too apically can result in infra-bony defects, periodontal pocketing, second stage complications, abutment connection problems as well as excess cement debris accumulation around implant restorations due to reduced access for cement removal. Implant sulcus depths should be not more than 3-4mm to prevent periodontal pocketing from occurring therefore it is important the implant are not placed to far apically because they can result in formation of deep probing depths around dental implant.[22]

In treatment planning dental implants, in addition to taking into consideration their positioning, factors such as that anatomy of the implant site as well as bone quality, quantity, width, length and height are also of paramount importance. The posterior maxilla presents with unique challenges such as a potential for reduced bone density, (type 4 bone) additionally, because of the location of the maxillary sinus in that location, loss of bone and pneumatization of sinus can occur in patients who have lost their teeth for a number of years. For patients that are requiring dental implants in the posterior maxilla, careful planning is required to address the limitations that are present in that location.

Sinus augmentation to augment the maxillary sinus and prevent dental implant placement that encroaches on the sinus cavity can be performed either utilizing a lateral window technique or utilizing osteotomes. When planning dental implant in the posterior maxilla region, a number of factors affect what technique that will be done. These include the number of dental implants planned, the height of bone that is present, the patient's level of tolerance to surgical procedures.

When there is less that 5mm of bone present between the sinus and the ridge, or when multiple implants are planned in the posterior area, the lateral window technique might be the more appropriate technique rather than the osteotome technique because of its ability to augment a larger area of the sinus. The osteotome technique that was developed by Summers has advantages to the lateral window procedure including less chances for post-operative complications or infections, reduced rate of perforation of the Schneiderian membrane, and less complicated surgical design. [25]

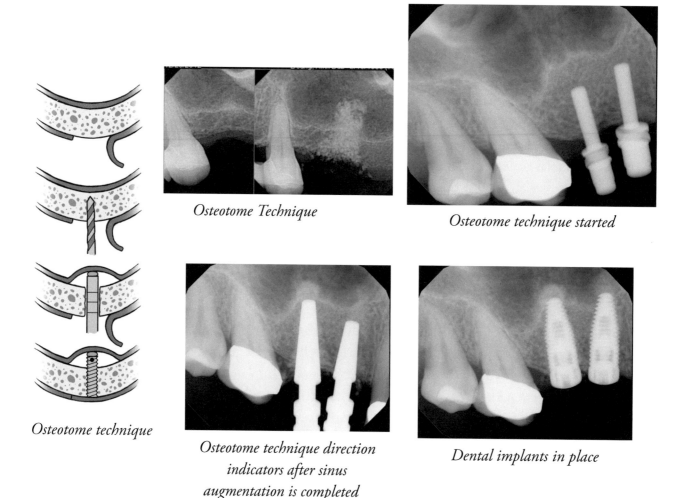

Osteotome Technique

Osteotome technique started

Osteotome technique

Osteotome technique direction
indicators after sinus
augmentation is completed

Dental implants in place

Studies conducted by Pal et al regarding comparison between osteotome sinus lift technique and lateral window sinus lift found both techniques were comparable in terms of post-operative pain and swelling, gingival status, bone height augmentation as well as stability of implant placement. [26]

Other techniques to help to create optimal dental implant sites prior to dental implant placement include soft tissue grafts to increase soft tissue around dental implants, socket preservation technique, and ridge augmentation of deficient ridges and they will be reviewed later in the book.

Chapter Summary 5: Site preparation prior and during Dental Implant placement.

1) Use of bone grafting procedures prior to dental implant placement is recommended for sites with less than 5mm of bone.

2) Particulate or block bone graft are used to increase bone volume. When bone augmentation is needed in both horizontal and vertical dimensions, then block grafts are typically recommended.

3) For implant success to occur, both having adequate bone volume as well as optimal dental implant position are criteria that are critical.

4) In classifying bone in a residual ridge a number of classification systems exist that categorize bone quality, quantity, volume and contours.

5) The Misch and Judy classification system classifies bone from a range of adequate to deficient. Category A refers to ridge with adequate bone of 5mm or more of bone in the buccal to lingual dimension with no need for bone grafting, while Category D refers to bone that is deficient and requires extensive bone augmentation.

6) In positioning implants in the apico-coronal dimension, the implant collar should be 2mm from CEJ of adjacent teeth if there is no recession and 3mm from the CEJ of adjacent teeth when recession is present. Excessive apical positioning of dental implants can lead to periodontal pocketing long term and formation of intra bony defects.

7) When sites in the mouth present with inadequate bone for dental implant placement, ridge augmentation procedures and ridge preservation procedures are recommended.

8) In the posterior maxilla, when inadequate bone height exists, sinus augmentation procedures or use of shorter implants are indicated.

CHAPTER 6

Bone and Soft tissue augmentation procedures prior to dental Implant placement

When teeth are treatment planned for extraction, a decision has to be made about if additional therapy is needed to maximize the chances of having sufficient quality and quantity of bone present for dental implant therapy. A procedure called socket preservation is usually treatment planned to be performed for extraction sites that will be receiving dental implants. It involves utilizing bone grafts with or without a collagen membrane following extraction with the goal of preserving the dimensions of the extraction socket after bone healing and maximizing bone fill and therefore optimizing adequate bone in three dimensions.

Ridge augmentation procedures are performed in sites which are already edentulous, but present with deficient bone in any or all dimensions for dental implant placement. Because teeth are extracted for different reasons that can include infection, bone loss, trauma and caries and for orthodontics, following initial extraction and bone grafting, a need for additional bone augmentation might still exist to ensure that adequate bone exists. In such cases, bone augmentation with either particulate or block graft may need to be completed prior to dental implant placement.

For adequate soft tissue contours to exist especially in the anterior area of the mouth the potential emergence profile for the ridge is evaluated. It should be harmonious with that of adjacent teeth in a vertical direction so that clinical crown height around adjacent teeth are not significantly different. According to Kazor et al soft tissue around a dental implant site should be convex, with adequate quality, quantity, color texture and biotype. When soft tissue is being augmented prior to dental implant placement over contouring by 2-4mm of tissue is required. Recession can occur post-surgery therefore over contouring can compensate for tissue loss. [22]

Assessing the emergence profile of a site requiring dental implants is important. If adequate bone exists, but a thin soft tissue biotype is noted that will not be adequate for preservation of health around dental implants as well as that might not be able to mask the underlying metal components of the implant restoration, soft tissue procedures to increase levels of attached tissue become necessary.

Gingival augmentation procedures such as free, pedicle, or sliding flaps might be indicated to increase soft tissue prior to or during dental implant placement if a one staged implant placement technique is being utilized. The two staged technique allows for additional soft tissue grafting during time of abutment placement, and prior to fabrication of the final dental implant restoration.

In treatment planning dental implants especially in the anterior maxillary area, the thin periodontal phenotype of the edentulous site is very important, and paying attention to the emergence profile prior to planning dental implants is essential. [27]According to Abramson et al, gingival recession increases in people with thin periodontal phenotypes compared to those with thick periodontal phenotype. Alveolar bone absorption tends to occur in the apical and lingual direction for people with thin periodontal phenotype, as a result, they are also prone to facial bone loss. Due to thinness of tissue, the titanium metal can often show through, assuming a graying color as it shows through in areas with recession. [28]

A thick biotype involves a gingival thickness of more than 2mm, while a thin profile involves one with less than 1.5mm of gingival thickness. A number of methods to measure gingival phenotype including use of periodontal probes, use of ultrasonics, as well as use of cone beam technology have all been utilized as means of measuring thickness of gingival tissue. However, one of the simplest and most predictable ways still involves placing a probe in the gingival sulcus. If the probe is visible at the free gingival margin then the tissue has a thin profile. If the probe is not visible the tooth has a thick gingival bio-type. [29]

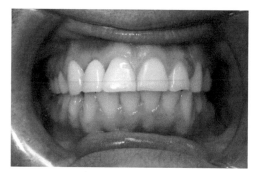
Thick gingival biotype

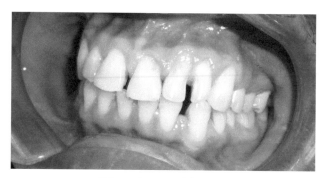
Thin Gingival biotype

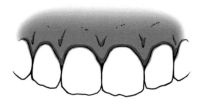

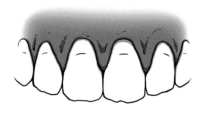

Types of gingival biotype

If it has been determined that a patient presents with thin periodontal phenotype, socket preservation techniques, ridge augmentation technique as well as soft tissue procedures to increase the thickness of tissue should be completed. Atraumatic tooth extractions are also extremely important for patients with thin biotypes because the goal is to preserve as much tissue as possible and avoid loss of bone that can occur during traumatic extraction. Immediate implant placement in people with thick biotypes is more predictable due to the ability of the tissue in the site to heal with minimal recession and ability for thicker biotypes to respond better to trauma.

Conversion from a thin to thick periodontal phenotype also involves soft tissue augmentation in addition to alveolar bone augmentation techniques. Use of soft tissue grafts such as sub-epithelial connective tissue graft, acellular dermal grafts, and modified roll techniques have been identified as methods to convert thin biotypes to thick biotypes. More recently, implant types have been introduced which use a pink collar instead of the metal colored implant collar in order to blend with adjacent gingival tissue and better mask the implant metal collar.[30]

Chapter 6 Summary: Bone and Soft tissue augmentation procedures completed prior to Dental Implants.

1) Teeth that are treatment planned for extraction and dental implants often require additional procedures to prepare the extraction sites for dental implants.
2) Procedures such as socket preservation which is done at time of extraction is helpful in preserving bone in the extraction socket.
3) Ridge augmentation procedures are performed in sites that are already edentulous that require additional bone.
4) Sites that are deficient in soft tissue can be augmented to increase keratinized tissue needed.
5) The goal during soft tissue augmentation is to over contour tissue by 2-3mm in order to compensate for recession that can occur post surgery.
6) Gingival biotype plays a major role in dental implant success. Thick biotypes have more than 2mm of gingival tissue while thin biotypes have less than 1.5mm of gingival tissue.
7) Sites that present with thin biotypes are more prone to recession and exposure of underlying titanium implant, therefore, techniques such as socket preservation, ridge augmentation, and atraumatic tooth removal techniques are essential when implants are planned in these sites. Sites with thick biotype are more resistant to trauma.
8) Gingival enhancement procedures such as sub-epithelial connective tissue grafts, grafting with acellular dermal grafts and modified roll technique are also helpful in increasing gingival tissue thickness and converting from a thin to a thicker gingival phenotype.

CHAPTER 7

Preparation and Steps for Dental Implant Surgery.

In preparing the patient for dental implant surgery, a prior evaluation to determine the type of sedation that the patient should be given is important. Typically, for less complicated cases, local anesthesia might be sufficient, for moderately complex cases, oral sedatives or nitrous oxide can be utilized, intravenous sedation and even general anesthesia may be necessary for more complex cases. Need for antibiotic prophylaxis is determined prior to implant surgery and some patients with pre-existing systemic conditions such as diabetics require this antibiotic coverage.

If oral sedation or prophylaxis is needed, prescriptions should have been dispensed prior to the day of surgery. The original protocol for sedation prior to implants according to Brannemark, Lekholm and Zarb indicate that ten milligrams of Diazepam be given the night before and another twenty to twenty five milligrams of Diazepam should be taken an hour before dental surgery prior to the surgical procedure.[31] Variations of use of oral sedation can be prescribed depending on the practitioner and most may choose to use a lesser dosage ranging from 5mg to 10mg on the day before and day of surgery.

Operatories are maintained in strict asepsis prior to the dental surgery. The light handles, are covered with sterile foil. The patient is also prepared for the surgery. Povidone iodine can be utilized to cleanse their face to ensure that the extra-oral environment closest to the implant site is also aseptic. Having the patient gaggle for thirty to sixty seconds with chlorhexidine is also very helpful in reducing intra-oral flora.

Once patient is adequately sedated, local anesthesia is administered. Typically, it usually depends on the number of implants that are being placed. When one implant is treatment planned, infiltration anesthesia is often sufficient, but when two or more dental implants are treatment planned, utilizing block anesthesia will be necessary. Following administration of local anesthesia, the bone in the areas should be sounded to determine the topography of bone. Access to the dental implant site is obtained and implant surgery is initiated.

Dental Implant Surgical placement utilizing a muco-periosteal flap:

When Muco-periosteal flaps are used, crestal incisions made slightly palatal or lingual on the ridge with mesial and distal release incisions made at line angles to the teeth adjacent to the edentulous site. A full thickness muco-periosteal flap is reflected to allow adequate visualization of the bone in the implant site. In the anterior area, the crestal incision is made towards the palatal aspect in order to allow for the preservation of most of the tissue to the facial, maximizing the chances to have an adequate amount of tissue to mask abutments. It also reduces recession and minimizes having excessively thin facial tissue after implant placement. It will also allow chances of having maximal blood supply to the flap as well as prevents scar formation. Papilla preservation flaps with mesial and distal releases made that does not include the interdental papilla can also be utilized in the anterior zone to prevent recession of tissue and dark triangles in the interdental papilla around restorations.

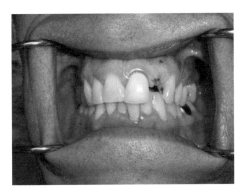

Anterior Immediate placement using mucoperiosteal flap

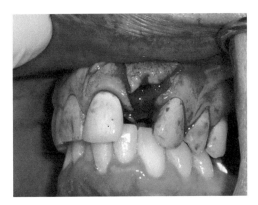

Anterior papilla preservation flap

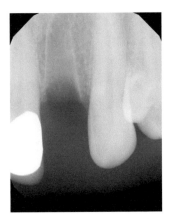

X-ray of extraction socket

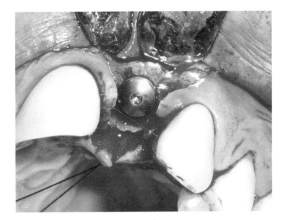

Dental implant placement

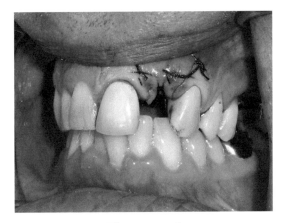

Flap sutured

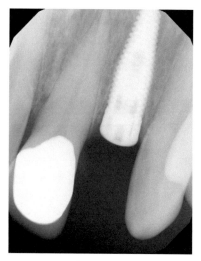

Dental implant x-ray

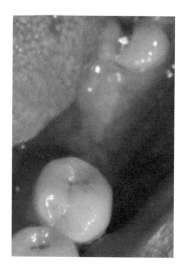

Posterior delayed implant placement

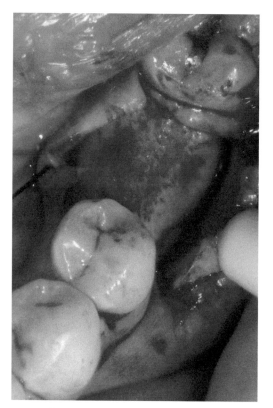

Papilla preservation mucoperiosteal flap

If a surgical guide is being utilized, it is then adapted to the appropriate location on the edentulous site and adjacent teeth. A surgical guide drill is placed through the access hole made in the surgical stent, and the implant surgery is initiated. The guide drill directs the initial location of the dental implant site. It is then followed by a series of twist drills and pilot drills under copious irrigation. If a completely fixed surgical stent is being utilized it is used for every drill placed with stops to ensure that the depth is also guided. Most stents used are only partially fixed so after the first drill is used to maintain precise positioning of dental implant site, and the remaining drills can be used in the established position.

Multiple x-rays are taken during the dental implant placement procedure, direction indicators are placed into the surgical site prior to x-rays to ensure adequate depth and angulation of the dental implant. Once adequate ostectomy is achieved for the implant site, the dental implant is then gently threaded into bone using an RPM of 35-50 Ncm. The initial bone to implant contact is a mechanical bond formed between dental implant threads and bone. Osteo-integration which is a chemical process occurs between the surface of a load bearing endosteal implant and bone tends to occur over a period of three to six months, depending on whether implant placement is in the maxilla or mandible.

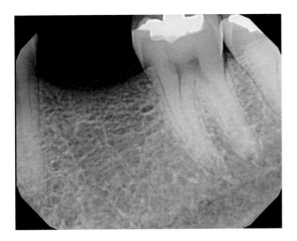

X-ray of surgical site

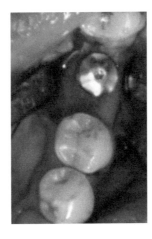

Healing abutment placed for non-submerged healing

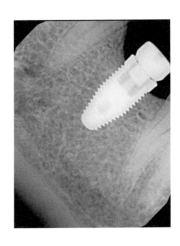

X-ray of dental implant in place

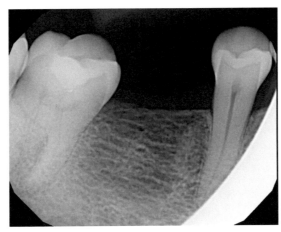

X-ray prior to non-submerged dental implant placement

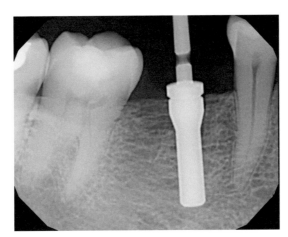

X-ray of direction indicator

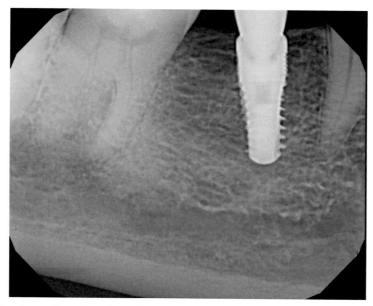

Implant placed with healing abutment for non-submerged healing

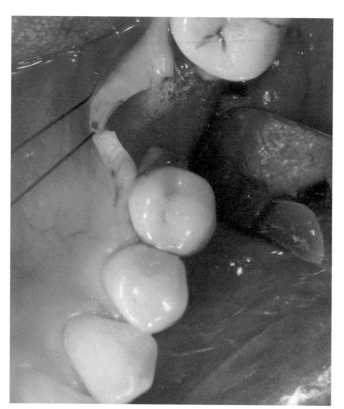

Mucoperiosteal flap

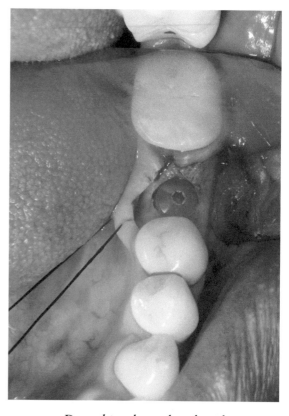

*Dental implant placed with
cover screw for submerged healing*

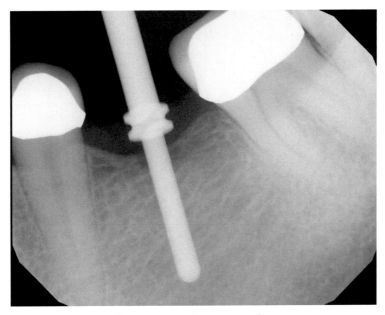

Direction indicator in place

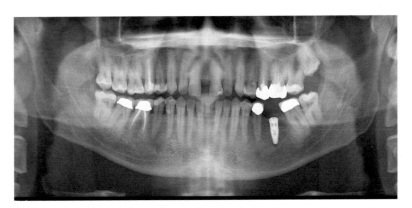

X-ray of dental implant placed with submerged protocol

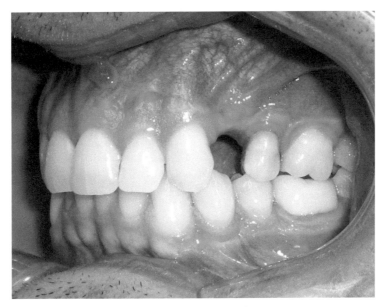

Site for dental implant placement

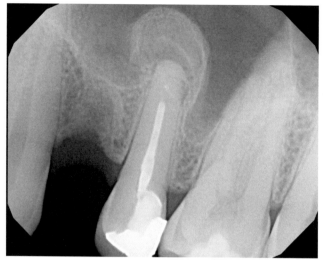

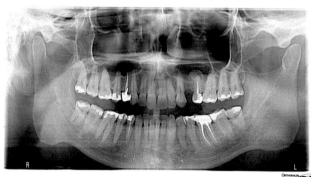

X-ray of Implant site

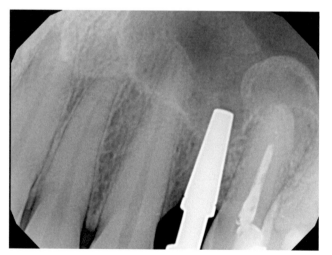

Direction indicator in place
for osteotome technique

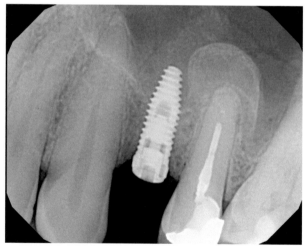

Dental implant in place

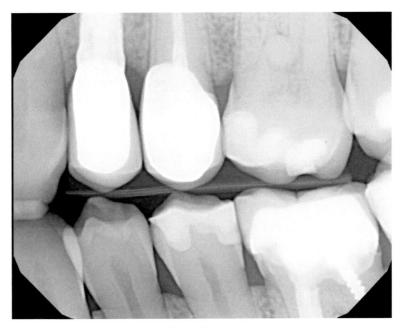

Dental implant restored

If no further bone grafting is needed at time of dental implant placement, a cover screw or abutment is inserted depending on whether a single stage or two stage dental implant surgical protocol is being utilized.

Dental Implant Placement Using Flapless technique:

Dental implants can also be placed using a flapless technique. The goal of this technique is to minimize trauma to the surgical site by not reflecting a full thickness flap, it also allows preservation of the soft tissue in the site, keeping the vasculature intact. There is also a reduction in surgical time, as well as better patient ease and less postoperative trauma. When utilizing the flapless technique, and utilizing guided technology, the goal is to work backwards. The surgical guides already fabricated prior to the day of surgery from CT scan x-rays is transmitted to be utilized in combination with CADCAM technology to generate surgical guides.

Following administration of local anesthesia, the surgical stent is placed, and the site for implant placement undergoes bone sounding and it is then marked with a guide drill. When standard diameter dental implants are being placed, a 5.0mm diameter tissue punch is used to get access to the underlying bone. When wider implant diameters then the standard 4.1 diameter is being placed, a 6mm tissue punch can be utilized.[32] Drills are used under copious irrigation with appropriate settings to prepare the ostectomy site, and preparation is confirmed using x-rays. The dental implant is then inserted into bone and locked at 30—50Ncm. X-rays are again taken to confirm accurate placement. [32] Flapless technique can also be performed using a scalpel.

Post operative instructions are given, and normal activity and oral hygiene resume almost immediately due to the minimally invasive nature of the procedure. The disadvantage of the Flapless technique involves the limited access that is available to underlying bone. There is also less visibility of anatomic landmarks, a potential for thermal damage and reduced ability to adapt soft tissue. It is also very technique sensitive so the recommendation is to utilize it after gaining proficiency at using mucoperiosteal flaps.[32]

Post-operative patient care after dental implant placement:

After periodontal surgery is completed. The patient is given a gauze pack to apply to the surgical site to control for any bleeding. Prescriptions for pain medication, usually involving Motrin 600-800mg or Tylenol #3 is given to patient. A prescription for an antibiotic, usually twenty one tablets of Amoxicillin 500mg, or Clindamycin if the patient is Penicillin allergic is also given to patient. A prescription for an anti-bacterial rinse is also given that is usually Chlorhexidine.

Post-operative instructions are given involving use of cold compresses to help prevent swelling. A soft bland diet which requires minimal effort with chewing is recommended, mastication on opposite side to the operated area, and avoiding hot fluids is also recommended. The patient is also advised to restrict physical activities for about three days to minimize post-operative bleeding.

If non-absorbable sutures are utilized, the patient presents in 7-10 days for suture removal and observation of the surgical site. If patient has removable partial dentures as temporary prosthesis the denture is relieved with a soft tissue conditioner or soft reline placed. The original protocol from Brannemark recommended not wearing the removable prosthesis for two weeks prior to the soft reline.[31] If a temporary bridge, or nesbite or other tooth borne temporary restoration is being utilized, then the restoration can be inserted immediately after the surgical procedure. The temporary restoration is adjustment prior to insertion to ensure it does not in any way encroach on the sutured dental implant site or have any occlusal interference with the opposing dentition.

After suture removal, the patient presents at five weeks for an additional post-operative check. The patient is examined clinically, and radiographs are taken to assess the progress of dental implant healing. Changing of relines and further adjustments to temporary restorations are also performed at this visit should they be necessary. For standard dental implants, osteo-integration occurs for three to four months in the mandible and four to six months in the maxilla. For accelerated dental implants surfaces, the healing time can be decreased to six weeks to two months. Following osteo-integration, the dental implants are then scheduled for second stage surgery, to uncover the implants, test osteo-integration and place a healing abutment which will allow adaptation of tissue in preparation for the future abutment and restoration.

Chapter 7 Summary: Preparation and Steps for Dental Implant Surgery.

1) Finalizing treatment planning utilizing panoramic, peri-apical x-rays and CT Scan.
2) Fabrication of Surgical guide.
3) Fabrication of temporary restoration.
4) Determining type of sedation anesthesia to use.
5) Scheduling of dental implant surgery.
6) Administering of anesthesia.
7) Incision and elevation of muco-periosteal flap.
8) Use of surgical guide for procedure.
9) Use of direction indicator and depth gauge during procedure to evaluate site preparation.
10) Taking of operative x-rays
11) Placement of dental implant and bone grafting material if needed
12) Closure of flap and post-operative instructions
13) Placement of temporary restorations on dental implant if immediate loading, adjustment of temporaries post implant placement for delay loading.
14) Suture removal in 7-10 days
15) Five week post-operative visit involving evaluation of surgical site as well as relines of temporary restorations if needed.
16) Scheduling of 2nd stage surgery.

CHAPTER 8

Dental Implant Uncovering and Second Stage Implant Surgery

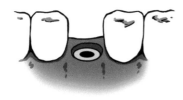

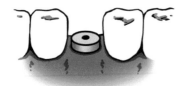

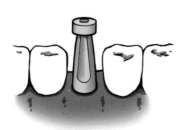

Dental implant uncovering, placement of healing abutment and impression coping

Following dental implant placement involving a submerged protocol, second stage surgery is performed to uncover dental implants and place a healing abutment that prepares the tissue around the implant for the restoration. When uncovering dental implants, a number of decisions are made based on the biotype of the tissue, the zone in the mouth, and the presence or absence of keratinized tissue and interdental papilla. These factors will affect the method that will be used for dental implant uncovering.

When the biotype is evaluated and it is noted that more than 4mm keratinized gingival tissue exists on an edentulous area, uncovering of the dental implant is done by excisional technique. When less than 4mm of keratinized tissue is noted, then an incisional approach is required. When an inadequate amount of keratinized tissue exists, grafting to increase the amount of tissue is recommended.

Excisional incisions involve use of either a tissue punch, scalpel or laser to excise tissue covering the cover screw in order to uncover the dental implant. An adequate thickness of keratinized tissue of at least more than 1mm has to be present all around the implant when the uncovering is completed with either the tissue punch or scalpel or laser.

When there is a need to increase keratinized tissue on the buccal aspect, an incisional technique utilizing a palatally advanced flap with incisions made on the palatal aspect and released with vertical incisions would allow the flap to be advanced forward and sutured in place. This will increase the amount of keratinized tissue noted on the buccal aspect.[34]

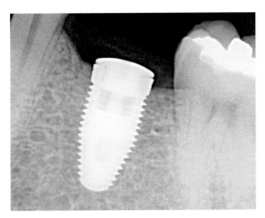

Dental implant

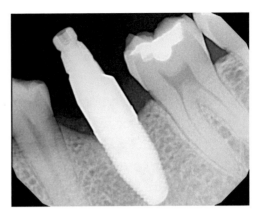

*Impression coping in place
for fabrication of custom
abutment and crown*

When there is an inadequate amount of keratinized tissue present, and the goal is to increase the tissue thickness, the roll flap technique can be used. This can involve a U-incision on the palatal aspect. The tissue becomes deepithelialized, and the tissue is moved to the facial to form a pouch, the tissue is then held in place with a sling suture, increasing the thickness of buccal tissue. [34]

Papilla preservation techniques during uncovering are also able to allow rebuilding of papilla around dental implants. When a significant amount of gingival augmentation is needed, free connective tissue grafts and pedicle grafts can be performed during second stage to ensure that there is an adequate amount of keratinized tissue around the dental implant. The connective tissue can be harvested from the palate, or maxillary tuberosity or acellular dermal grafts (Alloderm) can be utilized. When a pedicle is being used, tissue can be moved from the palatal aspect to the buccal aspect to allow for adequate thickness of facial tissue.[34]

Prior studies have shown that having an adequate band of attached tissue can be able to confer resistance to recession of gingival tissue and also prevent infection around dental implants. These studies have also noted the ability of increased width and thickness of keratinized tissue being associated with better implant success rate long term.[34]

Following uncovering of dental implants, healing abutments or temporary abutments can be placed. Cover screws are removed, and tests are done to assess the stability of osteointegration. While there is currently no definite method available to assess osteointegration methods that have been advocated include use of standard radiographs especially bitewing x-rays to evaluate crestal bone level, reverse torque test with torque of more than 20NCm indicating osteointegration, used of Mode analysis, use of periotest, as well as resonance frequency analysis (RFA) which uses small L shaped transducers tightened to the implant or abutment by a screw, to measure implant stability. But typically, standard radiographs and reverse torque test and periotest are methods most frequently used to assess osteointegration.

After healing abutments are placed, the implant is allowed to heal for two to three weeks. X-rays are taken after they are placed to ensure that the abutments are seated properly. Healing abutments allow soft tissue around the implant to form around it in preparation for impressions and fabrication of the permanent restorations.

Summary Chapter 8: Dental implant uncovering and Second stage surgery.

1) Second stage surgery is necessary to uncover submerged implants after osteointegration occurs.

2) Sites with thin biotypes will require incisional rather than excisional implant uncovering.

3) Sites with thicker biotypes that have adequate amounts of keratinized tissue can be uncovered with excisional techniques that remove tissue covering the dental implant with scalpels, tissue punches as well as with dental lasers.

4) Sites that have minimal keratinized tissue can be planned for uncovering with incisional techniques that increase attached tissue on the facial aspect as well as preserve tissue in the papilla area.

5) Sites that lack keratinized tissue should have soft tissue augmentation prior to receiving permanent restorations especially if they are located in the anterior zone.

6) After uncovering of the implants, the cover screw is removed and replaced with a healing abutment. X-rays are taken at the visit to ensure complete seating of the healing abutment.

7) While no specific way is currently in place to assess implant osteointegration, methods advocated include bitewing x-rays, reverse torque test, periotest, mode analysis, and resonance frequency analysis.

8) Impressions for permanent restorations usually occurs 2-4 weeks after dental implant uncovering depending on methods used.

CHAPTER 9

Selecting Dental Implant abutments and Impression techniques for Fixed Implant Restorations.

Following healing after second stage surgery has been completed with the submerged dental implant placement protocol, the next step is choosing abutments. A number of different options for types of abutments exist, two major categories of abutments are utilized; prefabricated and custom abutments.

Prefabricated abutments are machine made by dental implant companies to be placed on the corresponding implant type. The advantages of prefabricated abutments have to deal with the fact that since they require less components and less laboratory costs, they are also less expensive to place. They involve less visits in the dental chair so that receiving dental implant restorations are quicker. They are modified chairside utilizing the post and core concept, and impressions made after they are modified and sent to the laboratory. They are made of three major types of materials, pure titanium, titanium alloy as well as Zirconia abutments. [36]

Prefabricated abutments offer the advantage of durability as well as having fit accuracy because they are fabricated specifically for the dental implant type they are being utilized for. Their disadvantage lies in the fact that their design allows minimal abutment modification so that they cannot be typically used when there is a deviation of more than 15 degrees in angulation, nor do they fit the soft tissue profile as accurately because they are designed to fit the implant rather than the specific gingival architecture of patients.

Custom abutments are divided into custom cast abutments made by dental laboratory from wax-ups and CADCAM abutments which are custom abutments that are fabricated utilizing CADCAM technology to scan and fabricate the abutment. Custom cast abutments are more expensive because they require more components and a more elaborate laboratory process for their production. They have the advantage of fitting the soft tissue profile more accurately because they are designed to fit to the patient's gingival profile. They also are more modifiable in most parameters including emergence profile, thickness of abutment, finish lines and also overall contour.[37]

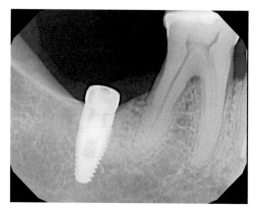
Dental implant after healing

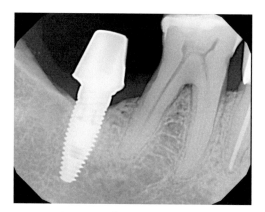
Custom abutment in place

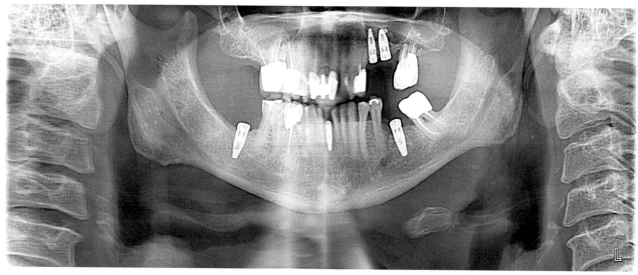
X-ray of dental implant post placement

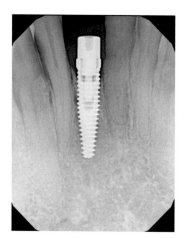
Anterior implant uncovered

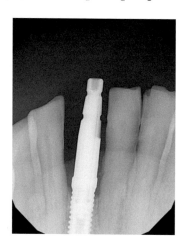
Impression coping in place

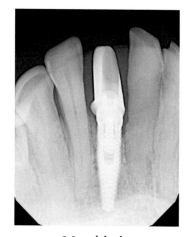
Mandibular anterior custom abutment

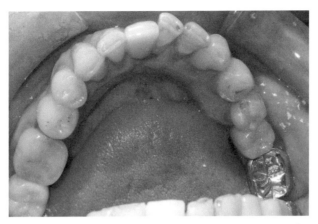

Anterior and posterior dental implants restored

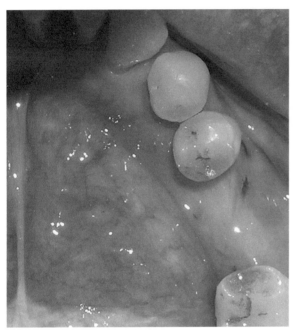

*Before implant placement
and restoration*

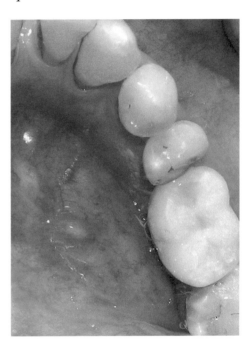

*Restoration of dental implant
with cemented crown*

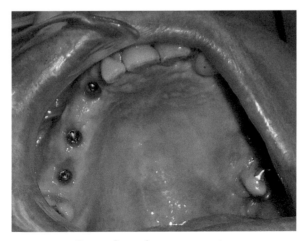

Dental implant uncovering

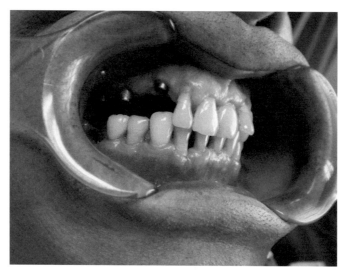

Healing abutments

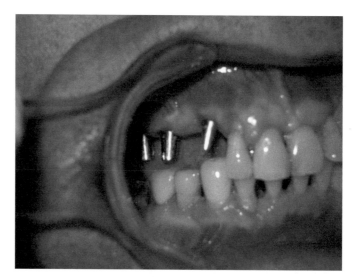

Custom abutment placement

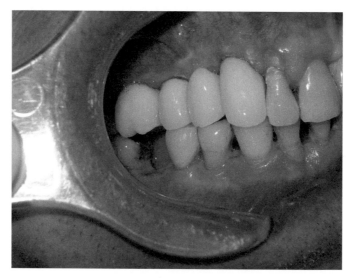

Cemented implant bridge

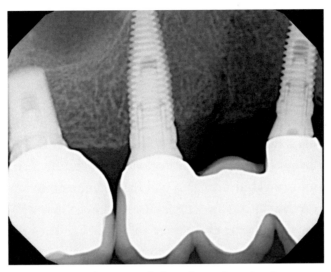

Xray of cemented dental implant bridge

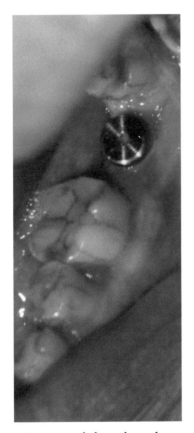

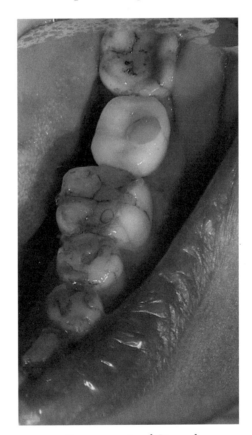

*Uncovered dental implant
with healing abutment*

*Screw retained Dental
implant crown*

CADCAM abutments combine advantages of both prefabricated as well as cast custom abutments, by reducing the number of components as well as simplifying the process of formation of custom abutments, they have made their production to be less labor intensive. In addition, they are very durable, and allow modification of abutments in emergence profile. They are also very accurate and have a predictable fit.

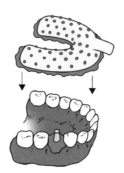

Advantages of CADCAM custom abutments in comparison to prefabricated abutments is that they offer more precision and accuracy, because they duplicate the soft tissue profile in the mouth, they also allow the advantages of prefabricated abutments by requiring minimal steps to final production of the abutment.

Clinical procedures for fabricating a custom abutment made in a laboratory involves utilizing an impression coping that is fixed on the dental implant, and utilizing either a closed tray or open tray technique to transfer the dimensions to forming an abutment that will fit the implant and gingival contours. The open tray technique involves removing the impression with the impression coping still inserted while the closed tray technique removes the impression first and then the impression coping is reinserted.

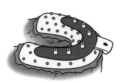

Closed versus Open
tray technique

The closed tray technique is usually recommended in areas in the mouth with limited access that will make it difficult to remove both the impressions and the copings at the same time. The open tray technique is regarded to be potentially more accurate than the closed tray technique because it removes all all the components at one time, which prevents discrepancies that could occur if the impression coping is not replaced back in exactly the same position.[38]

When the closed tray technique is being utilized, a standard impression tray can be utilized because the impression copings are removed after the impression has been removed. Many restorative clinicians find the closed tray technique easier to use and therefore use it more frequently. When an open tray technique is being utilized, a custom tray that has been modified to have access to remove the impression copings with the impression is needed or a modified impression tray with an opening made.[38]

Taking Impressions with the Open tray technique [39]:

1) *Fourteen days after uncovering of the dental implant, the gingival tissue is evaluated to ensure it is ready for impressions.*
2) *An alginate impression is made of the implant arch and then poured to create study models.*
3) *The study model is used to create a custom tray with an opening to allow visibility of the fixture mount. A stock tray with an opening made for the impression coping can also be used.*
4) *The healing abutments are removed and replaced with open tray impression copings.*
5) *The tray is tried in to ensure that the impression coping is visible through the opening.*
6) *A light bodied polyvinyl silicone material is injected around the impression copings, while the heavy bodied material is placed in the tray. Care is taken to make sure that the impressions coping extends out of the opening*
7) *After the impression sets, the screw in the impression coping is loosened. It is removed with the impression.*
8) *The impression is checked to ensure the accuracy of the margins.*

9) *Impression analog is firmly placed over the impression coping with care taken to prevent distortion of the impression.*

10) *A counter model is made from the opposing arch, a bite registration is taken, and the impression with the impression coping and analog inserted are sent to the dental laboratory for fabrication of a screw retained crown, or custom abutment if the restoration being placed is for a cement retained implant crown.*

Following uncovering of dental implants and placement of healing abutments, the tissue is allowed to heal for between ten days and fourteen days and then impression proceeds. Open tray technique gives the advantage of being able to allow accuracy even with divergent implants, it is not indicated for areas with limited opening, posterior areas of the mouth which are not accessible, and for patients have a gag reflex.[39]

Taking Impressions with the close tray technique can lead to a decrease in the level of accuracy because the impression is removed without the copings and following removal of the coping they are replaced back into the impression and sent to the laboratory. Failure to accurately place the copings in its exact position can result in discrepancies in the final restoration.

Taking Closed tray Impressions [39]:

1) *Healing abutments are removed after ten to fourteen days of implant uncovering.*

2) *The right size for the closed tray copings are chosen and placed on the implant fixture head.*

3) *Periapical x-rays can be taken to ensure complete fit of the impression coping the abutment if necessary.*

4) *A stock or custom tray can be tried to ensure it fits the arch.*

5) *A combination of light and heavy bodied silicone impression material is utilized for the impression. The light bodied material is injected around the impressions coping while the heavy bodied material is inserted in the tray. Care is taken to ensure that excessive light bodied material is not placed because it can affect replacing of the impression coping.*

6) *As soon as the impression sets, it is removed. The impression copings are removed from the mouth and reinserted into their position in the impression. The impressions should be checked to ensure that the tissue contours are captured in the impression and that coping placement is accurate.*

7) *Healing abutments are then replaced. Bite registrations, counter models, analogs and the impression are made and then sent to the dental laboratory.*

With the closed tray technique, there is an advantage in areas that present with limited access as well for patients with gag reflexes because the impression does not require as much inter-occlusal space as the open tray technique. For multiple dental implants, that are being restored at the same time, the open tray technique is more accurate because it does not require repositioning of multiple impression copings back into the impression.

Chapter 9 Summary: Selecting dental implant abutments and impression techniques for Fixed Dental implant restorations.

1) Two major choices are available when selecting abutment. These include Pre-fabricated and Custom abutments.

2) Pre-fabricated abutments include abutments that are made by implant companies to correspond to various implant sizes.

3) Types of prefabricated abutments include: temporary abutments, standard abutments, angled abutments, locator and ball type overdenture abutments, and zirconia abutments.

4) Custom Abutments involve abutments that are fabricated to fit specifications of patient's gingival tissue.

5) Custom Abutments can be either cast abutments that are made in dental laboratories or abutments that are fabricated utilizing CADCAM technology.

6) Advantages of custom abutments include ability of better and more accurate approximation to patient's tissue. They are also better able to be to better adapt to gingival tissue. They can also be modified easier to fit patient conditions because of the ability to vary thickness and contours of the abutment to better match individual patient conditions.

7) Prefabricated abutments are very durable and are less expensive than custom abutments and are less labor intensive.

8) Disadvantages of prefabricated abutments include that they are not as adaptable to individual patient tissue conditions, because they are fabricated according to specifications set by the implant companies to fit to individual dental implant sizes. They are however very durable.

9) Two techniques are available for taking impressions of abutments which include the open tray technique and closed tray technique.

10) The open tray technique is more precise because the impression copings are removed with the impression tray transferring their position from the mouth to the soft tissue model. With the closed tray technique reassembling the position of the copings in the impressions can introduce inaccuracy.

11) The closed tray involves fewer components, and is advantageous for taking impressions in patients in areas of the mouth with limited access or patients with restricted mouth opening. It is also helpful for taking impressions with patients with a gag reflex.

CHAPTER 10

Cemented versus Screw retained dental implant restorations

Dental implants that are supported by single crown or implant bridges can be either restored using screw retained restorations or cemented restorations. The major benefit of using screw retained restorations is their ability to be able to be retrieved without damaging the dental implants supporting them. Their use has become reduced as success rates of implants greatly improved to over ninety percent hence there is not as much a need to retrieve the implant restorations. [40]

Cement retained restorations offer a number of advantages including they have better occlusion and esthetics compared to screw retained prosthesis as well as improved passivity of seated cemented restorations. Because they lack screw access holes, they tend to enhance the strength of porcelain and acrylic resin and are therefore less prone to fracture.[40] Other advantages also include that cemented restorations involve less chair time, less components needed because there is not a needed to torque screws, as well as less overall cost.

Screw retained restorations still present as the restoration of choice in areas of the mouth where there is limited inter-occlusal access which would involve reduced abutment height and retention for cemented restorations. Because cemented restorations require abutment height of at least 5mm, and adequate surface area and taper, the retention gained from screw retained restorations in such areas can be able to offer superior retention because they require less space for the restorations compared to cemented restorations which have limited retention when there is inadequate space, taper or surface area.[41]

Most practitioners utilizing cemented restorations recommend initially cementing with temporary cements to ensure patient comfort and then utilizing permanent cements after a few months or when it has been determined that the restorations are comfortable for patients and that the restoration is overall successful.

A number of factors affect the retention of cemented restorations, these include abutment taper, abutment surface area and height, and the type of cement utilized. The amount of retention changes between when temporary or permanent cements are used, with permanent cements being more retentive. Cemented restorations are more esthetic than screw retained restorations and do not have un-esthetic access holes, they also are less prone to fracture as well as have a more passive seat of the restoration. Their disadvantages include that the cement might be difficult to remove and could cause oral hygiene problems. Use of permanent cements can make the restorations difficult to retrieve, and in areas of the mouth with limited inter-occlusal access, cemented restoration would not be the restorative choice because a minimum of at least 5mm of inter-occlusal space is needed for adequate retention of cemented restorations.

Screw retained restorations are required to be torqued to the manufacturers specifications, they recommend that screws are to be tightened to 50-75% of their yield strength to provide optimal retentive force.[40] Screw loosening is one of the major complications that can occur with screw retained dental implant restorations. According to studies, there is a 5% to 65% chance for screw loosening to occur, it is recommended that screws be torqued to 20-30NCm in order to prevent this from occurring[41].

Screw retained restorations are susceptible to vertical occlusal forces, and can also undergo screw loosening and fracture when excessive occlusal forces are present.

There is no statistical difference between screw retained and cemented restorations in terms of long term survival and success rate. The type of restoration to utilize is dependent on the practitioners preference and also the unique characteristic of the implant site such as inter-occlusal space, need for esthetics, and angulation of the implant and need for implant restoration to be retrievable [41].

Use of screw retained dental implant restoration are favored over cemented restorations when multiple teeth are being replaced with dental implants. The multi-unit dental implant restorations are splinted using screw retained restorations while single unit crowns and individual dental implant bridges are often cemented.

Chapter 10 Summary: Cemented versus screw retained dental implant restorations.

1) Fixed restorations for dental implants used to restore single crowns or fixed dental implant bridges can either be screw retained or cemented.

2) Screw retained restorations contain an access opening which makes them retrievable.

3) By being readily retrievable, screw retained restorations minimize damage to dental implants when restorations are removed.

4) Cement retained restorations offer a number of advantages including having a more passive fit for the restoration on the dental implant, and being more esthetic because there is no access hole present. They also allow better occlusal scheme and more strength with restorations.

5) Disadvantages of cemented restorations is that they are sensitive to the amount of taper present in the abutment, they also require a minimum abutment height of 5mm and require an adequate surface are. Therefore, an adequate inter occlusal space is needed for cemented restorations to be utilized.

6) In areas of the mouth with restricted access or limited opening, or areas with reduced inter-occlusal space, screw retained restorations are typically the best option for dental implant restoration.

7) Cemented restorations can be made retrievable by using temporary cements to restore the implants initially, and then use of permanent cement when the implants have been found to be successful.

8) Studies have found similar success rates were found for both cemented and screw retained restorations.

CHAPTER 11

Restorative Options for Edentulous patients (Overdentures and Fixed Restorations)

Dental implants were originally created to be utilized for completely edentulous patients who for various reasons could not tolerate wearing complete dentures often due to having a gag reflex. Over time dental implants have extended to replacement of single as well as multiple teeth with overall high success rates. A number of studies on edentulous patients were typically localized to the edentulous mandible where the presence of the tongue and other factors affected complete denture stability and retention. Most of the treatment goal in restoring edentulous mandibles have been geared towards improving overall function, and support of dentures. More recent studies have studied the edentulous maxilla, where other factors such as achieving esthetics plays a major role in addition to improved function to obtaining successful restoration of the edentulous patient. [42]

While most dentists who have just recently started placing dental implants will not be placing implants in completely edentulous patients due to the degree of complexity that these situations can present, it is essential that they are fully informed on how to treatment plan as well as to restore completely edentulous patients. Because as overall population is living longer, being able to offer restorative options that can be able to help enhance the quality of life for edentulous older patients is important.

During treatment planning edentulous patients, different restorative options exist. These include restoration with overdentures which are removable, restorations with fixed ceramo-metal implant restorations as well as use of hybrid prosthesis that combine both fixed and removable characteristics and are made of acrylic on a metal framework. Hybrid restorations have the ability to compensate for areas in the mouth with loss of bone and soft tissue while remaining fixed in the mouth.

For edentulous people that wear conventional dentures, they can encounter a number of limitations to quality of life such as difficulty with retaining dentures, problems with mastication as well as inability to tolerate the denture prosthesis. This is particularly prevalent in the mandible where the presence of the tongue and the floor of the mouth might make mandibular dentures mobile, and retention of dentures difficult.[42]

To better stabilize mandibular dentures, the use of dental implants have been advocated to be able to provide retention, and also preserve bone in the edentulous area. Over dentures are recommended for patients that present with complaint of dentures mobility without soft tissue discomfort [42]. The most minimal way to restore dental implants while significantly improving denture retention in to place two dental implants, and either restore with ball, clip or hadder bar type overdenture abutments. For patients with complaint of soft tissue impingement from dentures, use of hybrid prosthesis or fixed ceramo-metal restorations might be the better option. [43]

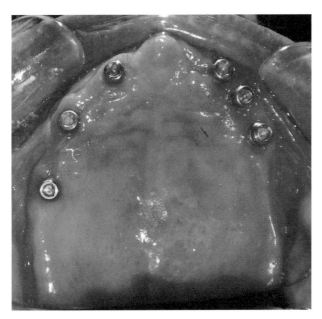

Maxillary overdenture abutments in place

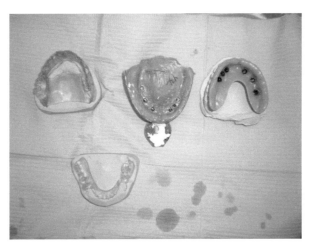

Surgical guide and over denture

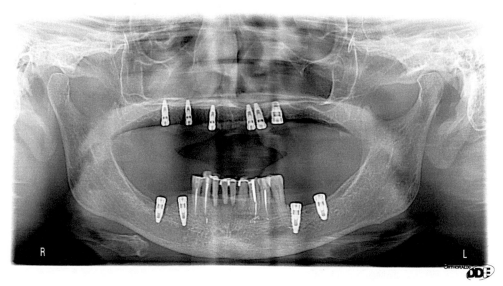

Dental implant for overdenture placement

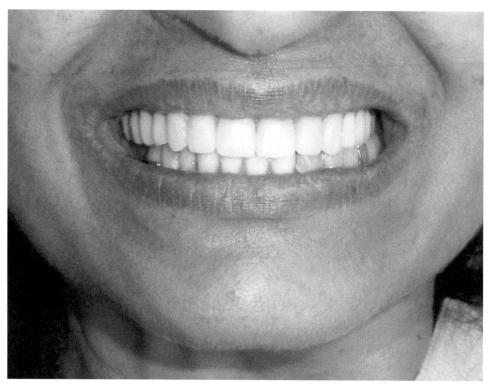

Overdenture in place

The advantages of overdentures include the reduced number of dental implants that are needed to retain the denture compared to fixed alternative making them highly cost effective. They are also easier to replace because their components are readily available from the manufacturer hence they can be repaired if damaged. In treatment planning overdentures, the patient's existing dentures can be utilized to function over the implants even further reducing the cost of dental implants. They can also be utilized in patients that have bone and soft tissue loss because a denture flange is usually present with the denture, it can be able to mask resorbed gingival tissue and bone.

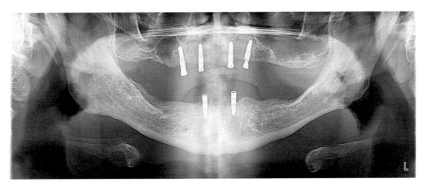

Minimalist approach to overdentures

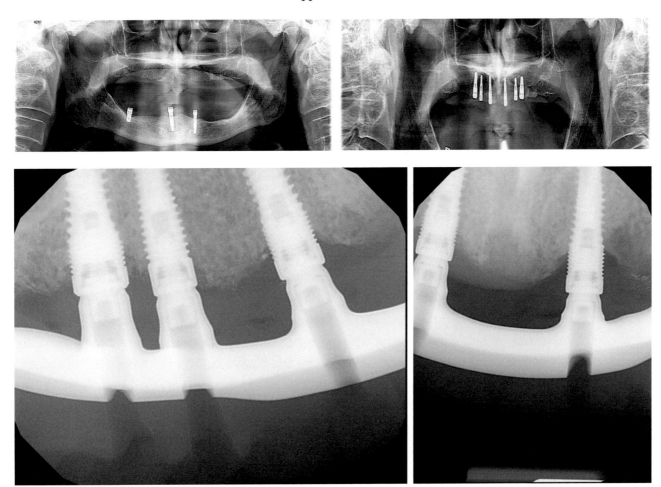

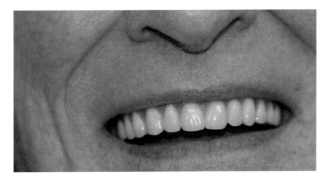

Hybrid prosthesis in place in patient's mouth

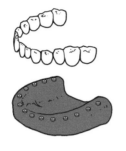

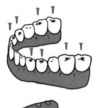

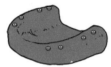

Fixed versus hybrid restoration

In the mandible, because the tongue and the floor of the mouth create problems with stability, most patients find dentures difficult to tolerate, and use of overdentures is highly recommended to improve denture retention. In planning mandibular over dentures, two to four dental implants can be utilized. While use of two implants is the minimalist yet effective way to restore implants with overdentures, use of four implants are even more retentive and can be used as individual overdenture abutments, or splinted with a bar for retention and stability. Use of bars to splint overdenture abutments are especially important for implants that might have divergent angulation and need to have the angulation corrected.

Use of overdentures involving two dental implants can be able to improve overall function for edentulous patient such as improved ability for mastication and speech by stabilizing the dentures during function. [44]

In treatment planning what implant restoration to choose for edentulous patients, a number of factors should be evaluated. These include the level of facial support that is present, bone or soft tissue deficiency present, the smile line of the patient, the upper lip length as well as the inter-occlusal distance present between the two arches. [43,45]

To evaluate the facial and lip support, the use of a patient's existing denture is indicated to evaluate for factors such as speech, function, denture relationship between both arches as well as overall esthetic concerns of the patient.[45] In addition, it will allow evaluation of the facial support to see whether or not improved support with either an overdenture with denture flanges for support, or use of pink porcelain in conjunction with fixed restorations might be necessary. It will also indicate if extensive bone and soft tissue grafting might be needed prior to dental implant placement. Evaluation of patient's facial profile is done before and after the denture is removed. The goal is to evaluate the level of lip support present. If the support is adequate then the patient can be recommended to have fixed restorations, if it is not adequate, it is important that the patient would be advised that they would need an overdenture rather than fixed option unless extensive bone grafting is performed prior to dental implant placement. [45]

Fixed dental implant restorations for edentulous patients can either occur using ceramo-metal bridges, individual crowns, or hybrid restorations. Hybrid prosthesis when used for edentulous patients offer fixed implant restorations that combine both the advantages of fixed restorations as well as able to compensate for missing periodontal tissue. They can be fabricated as acrylic screw retained restorations or can be cemented to abutments. Advantages of hybrid prosthesis in comparison to overdentures and ceramo-metal restorations is that they have reduced occlusal load compared to overdentures, they also are less expensive to fabricate than fully fixed ceramo-metal restorations, while at the same time they are still esthetic restorations that are fixed in jaws. [46]

Disadvantages of Hybrid prosthesis include food impaction occurring under the restoration, potential speech problems if not properly designed, and difficulty with oral hygiene for patients.[46] For patients that have complaints from discomfort from denture impingement on soft tissue, they offer the advantage over overdenture restorations of not being tissue supported, but derive their support from dental implants so that there is less chance of soft tissue encroachment. Hybrid prosthesis are usually fixed for patients but they can be removed by dentists. Their additional advantage is that they can be able to compensate for alveolar ridges where there is some resorption of the ridge and fixed ceramo-metal restorations would not present as a good option due to tissue loss.

The amount of implants needed to treatment plan for hybrid prosthesis varies, in the maxilla, usually 5-7 dental implants are recommended, in the mandible 4-6 dental implants are recommended for hybrid prosthesis. More or less implants can be treatment planned depending on the patient's oral condition. Hybrid prosthesis are recommended for highly esthetic areas, they are also the treatment of choice for patients that have increased inter-occlusal distance between the arches because they are able to compensate for loss of soft tissue. [46]

In designing the prosthesis, care must be taken to ensure that the framework that is utilized has a passive fit, so that the components of the restoration such as the screws, abutments as well as the acrylic fused to metal components do not fracture. Preliminary impressions are taken of both jaws, and they are mounted using a semi adjustable face bow transfer and occlusal jaw records. Impressions are made using either an open or closed tray technique. The abutments that are used can be splinted or the framework can be made on individual abutments. The metal framework is tried in the mouth and another impressions is made to complete the rest of the restoration that involves acrylic components.[46]

For patients that present with an adequate amount of tissue, and there are no restrictions such as financial concerns, fixed ceramo-metal restorations are an ideal choice for restoration of edentulous patients with fixed restorations. They are highly esthetic restorative options and also have an improved function and phonetics. They require an adequate amount of tissue support, and non excessive inter occlusal space of usually between 12-15mm. Typically, more cost is involved in terms of the components that is required for fixed ceramo-metal restorations. There is an increased number of dental implants compared to over denture and hybrid prosthesis.

A number of factors such as smile line, lip support, and patient esthetic concerns affect the choice of restorations to use and the need for ceramometal restorations.[46]. Fixed ceramometal restorations are the restorations that are the best option for restoring implants because they are the most esthetic option, they also transmit less force to dental implants compared to overdentures and hybrid prosthesis because their framework is more passive and as a result there is less pressure on the dental implant abutments. They also have had a long success rate for dental patients hence years after replacement with fixed restorations, patients present with overall satisfaction with the esthetics, function during mastication, as well phonation. [46]

Chapter Summary 11: Fixed dental implant restorations for edentulous patients: (Overdentures and Fixed Restorations.)

1) Restorative options for edentulous patients include overdentures, fixed ceramo-metal restorations and Hybrid restorations.

2) A number of conditions affect which restoration to utilize such as inter occlusal space, amount of loss of tissue, patient esthetic concerns, loss of alveolar tissue, patient smile line as well as lip length.

3) Evaluation of mounted occlusal record on semi adjustable articulator will allow for evaluation of alveolar ridge for any deficiencies, inter-occlusal relationship as well give information about what type of restorative options will be ideal.

4) Evaluation of smile line as well as lip length can be done by evaluating the patients existing dentures to determine how much of their teeth length is visible. This determines whether to have a denture flange would be necessary in which case an overdenture would be indicated versus fixed ceramo-metal restorations. Patient with longer lip length do not show as much their dentures when they smile which makes ceramo-metal restorations good options for them if adequate alveolar ridge dimensions exist.

5) In edentulous patient that have dental implants, when excessive alveolar deficiency exists, overdentures should be the restorations of choice, unless the patient is willing to under significant bone and soft tissue grafting.

6) Hybrid restorations are usually acrylic components over a metal framework. They are restorations of choice for denture wearers who indicated that they have soft tissue impingement from their dentures because they are completely implant supported and are fixed in the mouth. They are able to compensate for moderate ridge deficiencies by having acrylic denture components that mask the missing tissue. Their disadvantage is that the acrylic teeth can wear over time.

7) Fixed ceramo-metal restorations are highly esthetic restorations, their major disadvantage is their cost as well as the fact that they do not compensate well for deficiencies in alveolar ridge. While pink porcelain can compensate for mild to moderate deficiencies, patients with extensive deficiencies should be advised about removable alternative such as overdentures.

8) Managing patients' expectations in one of the most important part of restoring edentulous patients. While most edentulous patients would prefer to have fixed restorations due to their esthetics and improved function, being able to manage their expectations early for when this may not be an option is imperative to restorative success.

CHAPTER 12

Dental Implant Complications

While the success rate of dental implants have significantly improved over the past 40-50 years to levels above 90% in both the maxilla and mandible, failures can occur with dental implants which can be at time of placement, after placement or after the implants have been restored. The goal of this Chapter is to review the types of complications and failures that can occur with dental implants and recommended treatments that are available to address them.

Implant failures are can be caused by a number of factors, these can include patient factors such as type of bone quality and quantity the patient has in the implant site, patient oral hygiene practices, the presence of periodontal or endodontic infection in the implant site or close to it. Other factors that can contribute to dental implant failure can include oral habits such as bruxism as well as if the patient is a smoker. [47]

Dental implant failures can be divided into early and late implant failure. Early dental implant failures can occur weeks to months after dental implant placement and result due to failure of osteointegration to occur. This is due to factors that interfere with normal healing process and response and prevent the dental implant from becoming integrated.[48]

Predictors of potential implant failure include poor bone quality, chronic periodontitis in the implant site, systemic diseases that are uncontrolled, smoking, advanced age and implant location, with posterior maxilla having increased potential of failure compared to other areas of the mouth. Loss of implant integration, parafunctional habits as well as dental implant prosthesis that are not properly fabricated are also predicators of implant failure.[48]

Late dental implant failures involve pathologic processes that affect previously osteo-integrated dental implants. They occur after the implant is restored. The causes of late dental implant failure include loss of implant stability, contamination and peri-implant infection, trauma and occlusal overload. [48]Late failures can occur years after restoration of the implant so for patients the implant loss can be devastating.

Early dental implant failures are characterized by mild bone loss while late failures are characterized by moderate to severe bone loss. In the study by Yifat Manor et al, early failures occurred primarily due to failure of implants to osteo-integrate, 73.2% of their implants with early implant failures occurred because of lack of osteointegration while for implants in their late failure group, 32% occurred due to periimplantitis, 46.4% occurred as a result of occlusal overload, while 6.2% occurred due to dental implant fracture. [48]

Early dental implant failures are easier to treat than late failures because it is early in the implant process, and patients are more accepting of the option of dental implant replacement. Late failures by virtue of occurring later in the implant process after the implant has been restored already, makes that acceptance of the failure difficult for patients. Hence there is often a tendency on the part of both the patients and dentists to try to extend the duration of the implants in the mouth rather than removal and replacement of the dental implants.

While it is a worthwhile goal to retain implants, there is a recommendation made that the prognosis of the implants be evaluated prior to treating severely affected dental implants to ensure the implants have a major chance of responding to therapy rather than attempting therapy that might be futile in the long run especially in cases of extensive bone loss. By removing a failed implant earlier, the site can be grafted and patient presented with options such as dental implant replacement or conventional bridges.[48]

Other factors that can contribute to dental implant failures include clinician dependent factors as well as mechanical factors that are involved in dental implant prosthesis. Clinician dependent factors include site selection factors, case selection factors, implant design, implant number and spacing, and surgical technique of the clinician. Mechanical factors include occlusal overload of the restoration, problems with prosthesis design, and fractures of screws, abutments or dental implants. [47]

A number of clinical signs and symptoms are associated with failed or ailing implants. These include pain that can occur spontaneously or during mastication. Other signs of implant failure can include progressive bone loss that is noted on x-rays, periapical radioluscency around implant, mobility of dental implant in a horizontal or vertical dimension, progressive periodontal disease and inflammation noted around the dental implant . [47]

Dental implant failures caused by clinician dependent factors can be prevented by meticulous treatment planning, use of CT Scans and stents as well as all other key precautions that can be taken during treatment planning and also during dental implant placement.

Mucositis and periimplantitis are terms that have been used to describe periodontal disease that is occurring around dental implants. Mucositis refers to inflammation of the soft tissue surrounding dental implants. Periimplantitis refers to loss of bone and tissue around dental implants. The occurrence of periimplantitis is between 5-8%. [50]

In order to accurately diagnosis and treat mucositis and periimplantitis, it is important to perform a comprehensive exam involving probing depth measures, checking for bleeding on probing, as well as clinical signs of suppuration and mobility as well as using dental radiographs to evaluate bone loss around dental implants. Microbial analysis as well as culturing can be able to evaluate for species of bacteria that are associated with periimplantitis in order to provide an accurate diagnosis of peri-implantitis.[50]

Strains of bacteria that are associated with peri-implantitis include usually gram negative anaerobic bacteria, and spirochetes.[51] Bacterial strains including P. intermedia, P.gingivalis, A. Actinomycetemcomitans, B.

forsythus, T. denticola, P. Nigresens, F. nucleatum and P. Micros are often associated with lesions from peri-implantitis patients.[52] Mucositis has been found to be a precursor for peri-implantitis. Like gingivitis it is reversible, and therapy early can be able to prevent progression to peri-implantitis.

Treatment for Mucositis usually involves mechanical debridement with or without use of antibacterial mouthwashes and reestablishment of a good oral hygiene regimen. When appropriate therapy has been reinstituted, indications of mucositis such as bleeding on probing and inflammation can become reversed over time, halting progression to peri-implantitis.

Treatment for peri-implantitis involves non-surgical and surgical therapy. For mild to moderate peri-implantitis, use of mechanical debridement utilizing currettes, and adjunctive therapy such as antibiotics, antiseptics and chlorhexidine rinses are advocated. Use of lasers and also air abrasion are also recommended to affect the surface of implant threads removing contaminants on the implant surface and bacterial plaque allowing healing to occur around the implants.[52]

For implants that have advanced bone loss due to peri-implantitis, use of surgical therapy can be utilized to regenerate lost bone around dental implants using bone grafts and collagen grafts. Surgical flaps with bone graft and membranes are utilized. Overall many dental implant studies have shown improvement in clinical parameters such as bone fill, attachment level and reduction of bacterial colonies following guided tissue regeneration. [51,52]

Other potential causes of late dental implant failure can include dental implant fracture. Although it is rare (<6% occurrence rate) they can occur for a number of reasons including occlusal overload, non passive fit of implant prosthesis, biomechanical and physiologic overload of dental implant prosthesis, bruxism, clenching and oral habits, narrow dental implant diameter and bone resorption, and galvanic action of metals that were used in creating the dental implant prosthesis. [53]

Mechanical stress can occur on a dental implant prosthesis due to metal frameworks that do not have a passive fit causing screw loosening which is often a precursor of dental implant fracture. With multiple screw loosenings, the metal in the implant starts to fatigue and overtime dental implant fracture can occur. [53]

Parafunctional habits can be able to overload dental implants and are the third most common causative factors of dental implant fracture. [53]They should be addressed by therapy such as occlusal guards to prevent damage to dental implants.

Use of distal extensions as well as cantilevers should be avoided because they create occlusal load on the dental implants. On occasion when they are unavoidable, a reduction in the span of the cantilever should be incorporated into the prosthesis device to prevent possibility of excessive dental implant overload and dental implant fracture. [53]

Dental implants with smaller diameters are more prone to fracture especially in the posterior aspects of the mouth. Dental implants sizes that are 5 -6mm are found to be three times more resistant to fracture than implants that are 3.75mm in diameter. For the posterior areas of the mouth that are subjected to chewing forces, it is better to avoid very narrow diameter implants.[53]

In treating fractured implants, the treatment of choice is removal of the implant and replacement in the future with another implant. Other methods of treating dental implant fractures include altering the implant prosthesis to fit to the osteo-integrated fractured implant, or altering the fractured part of the dental implant and making a new prosthesis to fit to the altered implant dimensions. [53]

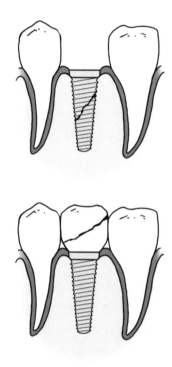

Dental Implant Fractures

Chapter 12: Summary on Dental Implant Complications:

1) Dental implant failures can be caused by a number of factors including patient dependent factors, clinician dependent factors and also biomechanical factors.

2) Two types of dental implant failures occur, Early and Late Fractures.

3) Early failures result from failure of dental implants to integrate.

4) Late failures result after dental implant restoration.

5) Factors affecting Early dental implant failure include poor bone quality and quantity, chronic periodontitis, uncontrolled disease, smoking, overheating of bone, and lack of primary dental implant stability.

6) Factors causing late dental implant failures include periimplantitis, Occlusal trauma and overloading of prosthesis.

7) Implant failures can be diagnosed by clinical symptoms such as pain on mastication or spontaneous pain, suppuration, and progressive bone loss on x-rays and mobility.

8) Mucositis refers to inflammation of soft tissue around implants, it is reversible.

9) Periimplantitis refers to loss of bone and tissue around dental implants.

10) Bacterial strains associated with periimplantitis are usually similar to those found in Advanced periodontitis and include gram negative anaerobic bacteria and spirochetes and include strains such as P.intermedia, P. gingivalis, A.actinomycetemcomitans, B. Forsythus, T.denticola, P.nigrescens, P.micros and F. nucleatum.

11) Treatment of Mucositis includes mechanical debridement with or without antimicrobial rinses and reestablishment of good oral hygiene regimen.

12) Treatment of Periimplantitis involves nonsurgical and surgical therapy. Nonsurgical therapy involves scaling and root planning in combination with adjunctive therapy such as antibiotics, antiseptics, chlorhexidine, lasers and use of air abrasion to remove contaminant from the surface of dental implants allowing healing.

13) Surgical therapy involves use of bone graft and membranes and laser therapy to regain bone around dental implants especially around dental implants with severe bone loss.

14) Mechanical stress in dental implant prosthesis can lead to implant fracture. Non passive implant prosthesis can result in multiple screw loosening which over time can lead to metal fatigue, and dental implant fracture.

15) Bruxism and other parafunctional habits, excessive span of cantilever and distal extension of implant prosthesis can also lead to dental implant fracture.

16) Avoiding very narrow implants in molar areas can help to reduce chances of implant fracture.

17) In treating dental implant fractures, the fractured dental implant is treated usually by removal.

CHAPTER 13

Dental Implant Maintenance

Following placement and restoration of dental implants, the goal becomes how to maintain the dental implants so that they continue to function long term. This involves a well defined implant maintenance regimen, where the condition of the dental implants are monitored routinely, and the components of the dental implant system are cleaned and adjusted to allow optimal function and health.

While maintenance of dental implants vary depending on the type of implant restoration being utilized, there are a number of key components that are required to ensure appropriate maintenance of implants long term. The frequency for dental implant maintenance can vary depending on the type of prosthesis as well as the specific characteristics of the dental implant site. The overall recommendation is that dental implants should be monitored on a six month schedule unless the implants have specific conditions that require more frequent monitoring such as bone loss, in which case the maintenance schedule should be increased to three to four months. [54]

Other maintenance recommendations include that the maintenance schedule can be for every three months after restoration of implants for the first year, and every six months afterwards based on if there are signs of periimplantitis, and if signs exist then the schedule should continue every three months. [55] The choice of what schedule to utilize is at the discretion of the dentist's philosophy regarding maintenance.

In general implant maintenance would involve a medical history review, comprehensive examination to assess the condition of the periodontal tissue around implants to ensure that there are no signs of inflammation such as bleeding on probing present, bacterial plaque and calculus deposits and suppuration present. Probing depth measures are completed including probing depth and attachment measurements around dental implants. X-rays are also taken that allow evaluation of bone around the dental implant for potential progressing bone loss.

Other parts of the maintenance visit would involve evaluation of the dental implant prosthesis, cleaning of the dental implant prosthesis, and repair, replacement or adjustment of any part of the dental implant restoration that has become impaired. If the dental implant shows signs of peri-implantitis, then the required therapy should be completed. Therapy for periimplantitis can involve non-surgical or surgical therapy depending on the progression of the disease.

Oral hygiene should be assessed and instructions given on how to continue to maintain the periodontal health around the prosthesis. Oral hygiene devices used at home should be safe to use on dental implant surfaces, and includes soft tooth brushes, interdental brushes, end tuft brushes and also multiple types of dental flosses which are designed to remove plaque around dental implant prosthesis[55]

In evaluating dental implants clinically for signs of inflammation. Clinical findings should be confirmed by completing a comprehensive periodontal exam assessing probing depth, attachment levels, and mobility around the implants and utilizing dental x-rays to confirm is periimplantitis is present. [55]

If mobility exists around a dental implant as a whole, it has failed and should be removed. The patient should be given options including replacement of the dental implant, fixed conventional restorations or removable prosthesis. Usually when clinical signs of periimplantitis exist they are confirmed by radiographs and manifest as bone loss on the x-ray. Implant mucositis is an inflammatory lesion that is localized to soft tissue without progression to bone loss. Periimplantitis occurs when the inflammatory lesion extends to cause bone loss around a dental implant.[55]

Implant restorations can be removable, or fixed with screws or cement. For removable restorations such as over dentures, during the maintenance visit, the restorations should be checked for stability and retention. Components such as clips that need to be replaced to improve retention should be replaced to ensure their continued function. Removable dentures should be cleaned extra-orally using cleaning agents. [54] The tissue around the abutments should also be checked to ensure that they are no major signs of inflammation such as bleeding on probing, and plaque and calculus build up should be removed using plastic curettes.

Occlusion on dental implants should be evaluated to ensure that they are not suffering from overload due to loss of support as the ridge resorbs around overdenture restorations. The retentive components that might lose retention as the bone changes should be replaced to ensure their continued function. [54]

Screw retained prosthesis have restorative materials such as acryllic over retentive screws that can become worn or lost over time and should be checked to see if replacement is needed. The retentive screws should also be checked to see if they are loosened. Frequently loosened screws can occur when the framework of the dental implant prosthesis is not fitting properly, or when there is excess occlusal load. If the loosening of screws is due to occlusal load that is excessive, occlusion should be checked and adjusted and the screws tightened or replaced if needed. [56]If the framework is ill fitting the restoration should be remade.

In evaluating implant retained prosthesis a number of factors are important such as the condition of the prosthesis, evaluation of screw retention and also cementation of the cemented restorations, evaluation of abutment, status of soft tissue as well as the radiographic findings. [56]

Loss of cement in single implant restorations is rare, the major complication that occurs with cemented restorations is failure to seat the dental implant prosthesis properly resulting in poor marginal seal and cement exposure that can cause inflammation of soft tissue. Removal of excess cement and re-cementation when necessary should be performed.[56]

Other complications that should be evaluated involve abutment loosening over time due to masticatory forces leading to development of a gap between the abutment and dental implants. It usually occurs in people with parafunctional habits or excessive occlusal contours and contact. The abutment should be removed and reinserted and adjustments made to the occlusion on the dental implant prosthesis if excessive occlusal contours are present. For patients with parafunctional habits, occlusal guards should be fabricated to protect the dental implant prosthesis.

X-rays should be used to assess dental implant marginal fit and the presence of bone loss. If bone loss is present, the cause should be determined. It can be caused by occlusal overload or by bacterial plaque. Excessive occlusal factors that can cause bone loss include history of parafunctional habits such as bruxism and clenching, history of breaking of dental implant substructure or screw loosening, too few implants replacing missing teeth, and excessive cantilever span. [56]

Presence of bone loss that is related to bacterial infection occurs for a number of reasons such as poor oral hygiene, loss of cement retention and tissue micro-gap between dental implants components, presence of inflammation, exudate and proliferation of soft tissue. Treating of the inflammation would involve removal of plaque and calculus using plastic curettes and air abrasion techniques rather than stainless steel curettes. Use of ultrasonic scalers are contraindicated around dental implants.[56]

Other implant complications that can be addressed during maintenance can involve frequent retentive screw loosening, which overtime can result in metal fatigue and eventual dental implant fracture. When an implant is fractured, and the fracture is significant, the retained fractured component can either be buried or removed. Implant removal involves a complicated process that involves use of a trephine to remove bone around the dental implant. This process can lead to potential bone defects in the area, so in rare cases of proximity to vital anatomic sites, the fractured implant can be buried rather than removed.

Evaluation of the prosthesis as well as the dental implant to ensure health and optimal function is the key reason for dental implant maintenance. In cases when progressing bone loss is noted on dental x-rays, decisions have to be made on how to address the condition. For early and moderate periimplantitis, non surgical therapy involving scaling and root planning using plastic instruments as well as air abrasion techniques in combination with chemical therapeutics such as chlorhexidine, antiseptics, and antibiotics can be utilized. Dental lasers can also be utilized.[52]

Affecting the surface of the implants is an important component of bacterial decontamination especially for rough surfaced and coated implant surfaces that can accumulate bacterial plaque due to the surface characteristics compared to smooth surfaced implant surfaces, affecting the surface with chemotherapeutic agents is of paramount importance to treating the dental implant surface. [55,56]

For dental implants with advanced periodontitis use of bone grafts and membranes to regenerate bone as well as laser therapy to regain bone is also advocated. Soft tissue around dental implants can also be affected resulting in tissue proliferation as well as tissue loss in some instances. Gingivectomy procedures as well as gingival flap are used to reduce excess tissue and allow maintenance of gingival health.[56]

Implants that show signs of periimplantitis and soft tissue complications should be monitored more closely after the condition is treated. The need for closer observation is needed to prevent progression of the condition as well as evaluate effect of healing long term. Dental implant maintenance is extremely important to overall dental implant continued success, and the ability for patients to understand that need for continued care for their dental implants after restoration will affect the future health and function of their implants.

Summary of Chapter 13: Dental implant maintenance

1) Dental implant maintenance is essential to long term health and function of dental implants and their restorations.

2) Key aspects of the maintenance visit include a review of medical history, a clinical exam evaluating for signs of inflammation such as redness and bleeding on probing. A periodontal exam evaluating probing depth, attachment level as well as mobility around dental implants. X-rays are taken to confirm clinical signs present.

3) Occlusion is also evaluated to identify and address excessive occlusal load that can happen from hyper-occlusion or from parafunctional habits such as bruxism. The dental implant prosthesis is also evaluated to ensure precise fit and continued function. Oral hygiene is also reviewed during the maintenance visit and use of oral hygiene dentrifices that do not alter the dental implants are recommended.

4) The maintenance schedule can be every six months or every 3-4 months depending on the overall health of tissue around the dental implant.

5) Mucositis refers to an inflammatory lesion that is contained within soft tissue around dental implants. It does not extend to bone. It can be diagnosed clinically by the presence of redness or bleeding on probing around dental implants.

6) Periimplantitis refers to an inflammatory lesion that extend to cause loss of bone around dental implants. The clinical signs noted can be confirmed with dental x-rays for a diagnosis to be made of Periimplantitis.

7) Occlusion is checked during the maintenance visit. High occlusal contacts can be reduced with occlusal adjustment and parafunctional habits can be addressed with occlusal guards.

8) When Scaling and root planning is performed around dental implants to remove plaque and calculus, use of plastic curettes are recommended. Ultrasonics are contraindicated around dental implants.

9) In treating mild to moderate periimplantitis non surgical therapy with scaling and root planning using plastic currettes, air abrasion in combination with chemical therapeutics are advocated removed plaque from the dental implant especially for rough surface implants. Use of dental lasers are also indicated to detoxify dental implant surfaces.

10) For patients with Advanced periimplantitis use of periodontal surgery and bone grafts are advocated.

11) In evaluating overdenture prosthesis, their retentive components should be checked for retention and stability. The components should be replaced if there is need for added retention.

12) For fixed screw retained dental implant restorations, the screws should be checked to ensure adequate retention, loose screws should be replaced and tightened. Restorative materials covering the screws should also be replaced if they have become worn or are lost.

13) For cemented dental implant restorations, they should be checked for marginal fit, and any excess cement should be removed to prevent causing periimplantitis long term.

CHAPTER 14

Conclusion

Dental implants have proven to be a remarkable discovery which has truly transformed dentistry as a whole. They have continued to increase in prevalence and overall efficacy over time. As their success rates in patients have increased, so have their popularity. The advent of CT Scans and CADCAM stents have increased the overall precision of dental implants allowing them to be performed with accuracy, safety, and with minimal discomfort and significantly reduced recovery time for patients.

The emphasis on implant placement today is restorative driven. Which means that dental implants are placed into sites which will result in good restorative outcomes as well as that present with adequate bone for optimal surgical placement. This requires that procedures such as bone augmentation, soft tissue augmentation and sinus lifts would be planned to ensure that implants are placed into sites that can be able to support dental implants.

The previous surgical guided implant placement involved the placement of implants into sites that have bone and then correcting any discrepancies that might have been caused during the implant restoration phase. A number of technological advancements have been responsible for the change of emphasis including the increased use of CT scans in dentistry, and the increased use and availability of regenerative materials including allogenic bone blocks, collagen reinforced and titanium reinforced membranes and pericardial membranes all of which are available for use in augmentation of potential dental implant sites.

Based on the technology that is available today, dental implants can be placed with the end results in mind. Using CT guided technology as well as CADCAM stents, the placement can occur into sites with adequate bone support, as well as in areas with optimal position for restorations. It has also significantly reduced errors that can occur by being able to identify anatomic structures such as location of nerves and maxillary sinus, so that implant placement does not impinge on vital structures. The wait time to receive dental implant restorations have been significantly reduced with capability of immediate loading, use of flapless technique as well as implants that are designed to better mimic gingival tissue, improving esthetics.

The goal of this book was to provide a comprehensive guide on treatment planning and implementing dental implants as part of a dental practice. The goal was to also review various surgical advances such as use of flapless technique, different types of stents available, delayed versus immediate dental implant placement and restoration, as well as techniques for uncovering dental implants. It also reviewed types of impression techniques available and the reasoning behind which one to utilize.

In choosing how to restore implants, it provides a review about when to choose screw retained versus cemented fixed implant restorations, and also reviews treatment planning of edentulous patients.

Despite the success of dental implants being at one of their highest levels, a number of complications can occur. These failures can be due to early failures during dental implant placement or as late failures after dental implant restoration. Early failure usually occur due to patient related factors such as deficient bone density and quality, and infection such as periimplantitis. They can also occur due to clinician related errors and contamination during implant placement while late failures can occur due hyper-occlusion, parafunctional habits, periimplantitis and problems with implant design.[48]

As the precision for planning for dental implants has improved a number of clinician related complications can be avoided by use of surgical guides and CT scan x-rays to evaluate bone quality as well as if there is adequate quantity of bone for dental implant placement.[57]

The importance of periodontal maintenance in preserving the longevity of implants in the mouth cannot be overstressed. The goal has been preventing periimplantitis by disruption and removal of bacteria from around dental implant surfaces as well as implementing good oral hygiene measures and debridement around dental implants to prevent bacterial accumulation. Studies have noted that there is increased bone resorption found around dental implant fixtures in edentulous patients with poor oral hygiene in comparison to those with good oral hygiene.[57] With dental implant maintenance, the goal is keeping the tissue around dental implants healthy just as with teeth so that they can be able to last for a long time in the mouth.

References

1) Handelsman M. Surgical guidelines for dental implants placement. British Dental Journal 2006;201.pp139-152.

2) Ticher et al. "The first implant" Protocol for the GP Part1, Treatment planning. Dentistry Today August 2011.

3) DeSouza KM et al. Types of Implant Surgical guides in Dentistry: A Review. Journal of Implantology 2011, 38(5): 643-652.

4) Pal US et al. Role of Surgical stents in determining position of Implants. National Journal of Maxillofacial Surgery.2010. Jan-Jun, 1(1):20-23.

5) Hinckfuss S et al. Effect of Surgical guide design and Surgeon's experience on accuracy of Implant placement. Journal of Implantology,2012 vol 38(4):311-323.

6) Jivraj et al, Treatment planning of Implants in the posterior quadrants. British dental journal 2006 (201): 13-23.

7) Shenoy VK. Single tooth Implants. Pretreatment considerations and pre-treatment evaluation. Journal of Interdisciplinary Dentistry 2012;2:149-157.

8) Buser D.et al. Optimizing esthetics for Implant restorations in Anterior maxilla: Anatomic and Surgical considerations. International Journal of Oral and Maxillofacial implants 2004;19(Supplement):pp43-61.

9) Bornstein M. Systemic Conditions and Treatments as risks for Implant therapy. International Journal of Oral and Maxillofacial Implants 2009. 24(Supplement): pp12-27.

10) Juodzbalys et al. Mandibular third molar impaction. Review and literature and a proposal for Classification. Journal of Oral and Maxillofacial Research 2013. April-June;4(2): E1.

11) Sugerman P et al. Patient selection for endoosseous dental implants. Oral and systemic considerations. International Journal of Oral and Maxillofacial Implants 2002;17:191-201.

12) Althassani A. Inferior Alveolar Nerve Injury in implant dentistry: Diagnosis, Causes, prevention and management. Journal of Oral Implantology 2010. 26(5):402-407.

13) Juodzbalyz G. Clinical and Radiographic classification of Jawbone anatomy in Endoosseous Implants, Dental Implant treatment. Journal of Oral Maxillofacial Research 2013. 4(2):1-17.

14) Greenstein et al. Clinical Recommendations for Avoiding and managing surgical associated complications associated with Implant Dentistry: A Review. Journal of Periodontology 2008;79:1317-1329.

15) Balshi TJ et al. A Retrospective comparison of implants in the Pterygomaxillary region: Implant placement with 2 staged, single staged and guided surgical protocol. International Journal of Maxillofacial Implants 2013;28:pp184-189.

16) Orentlicher G et al. Computer guided Implant surgery. Indications and guidelines. Compendium of Continuing Education;Nov/Dec 2012;33:10:pp720-733.

17) Orentlicher G et al. Computer Guided Planning and placement of Dental Implants. Atlas of Oral and Maxillofacial Surgery Clinics of North America;20 (2012):pp 53-79.

18) Flanagan D. Flapless Dental Implant Placement. Journal of Oral Implantology2007;33(2):pp75-83.

19) Salama H et al. The role of orthodontic extrusive remodeling in enhancement of soft and hard tissue profiles prior to Dental Implant Placement. A systematic approach to management of Extraction site defects. International Journal of Periodontics and Restorative Dentistry 1993;13:pp313-333.

20) Chu SJ et al. Subclassification and Clinical management of extraction sockets with labial dental alveolar defects. Compendium of Continuing Education. July/August 2015; 36(7):pp516-525.

21) Greenstein G et al, Immediate implant placement technique. Dentistry Today. May 2014. pp 1-12.

22) Kazor et al. Implant Plastic Surgery: A review and rationale. Journal of Oral Implantology 2004;30(4):pp240-254.

23) Lekholm U and Zarb CT. (1985) Patient selection and preparation (In tissue Integrated Osteointegration):pp199-209. Chicago, Illinois: Quintessence Books.

24) Misch CE et al. Classification of Partially edentulous dental arches for Implant Dentistry. International Journal of Oral Implantology 1987:4:pp7-13.

25) Summers R. A new concept of Maxillary Implant surgery: The Osteotome technique. Compendium of Continuing education 1994, Feb 15(2): pp152-156.

26) Pal US et al. Direct versus Indirect Sinus lift procedure. A comparison. National Journal of Maxillofacial surgery 2012. Jan-Jun 3(1):pp31-37.

27) Pallaci P et al. Soft tissue enhancement of Dental Implants. Periodontology 2000;47(2008): pp113-132.

28) Esfahrood ZR et al. Gingival Biotype a Review. General Dentistry 2013(7):pp14-17.

29) Abraham S et al. Gingival Biotype and Clinical Significance: A Review. Saudi Journal of Dental Research;5(11)2015: pp3-7.

30) Murphy KG et al. A report of three cases from an ongoing prospective clinical study on novel pink biomimetic implant system. Compendium of Continuing Education 2016(Supplement);37(2):pp1-11.

31) Brannemark PI et al (1985). Introduction to Osteointegration.(In Tissue Integrated Osteointegration) Chicago Illinois: Quintessence books.

32) Yong LT. Minimally invasive surgical placement of Non submerged Dental implants. A case series report. Evaluation of Surgical technique and complications. Journal of Oral Implantology 2011;37(4):pp579-587.

33) Sutchetcha A et al. Optimizing Esthetics in Second stage Dental Implant surgery: Periodontist's ingenuity. Journal of Dental Implants 2014;4(2):pp170-175.

34) Azar DE. Uncovering technique: Emphasis on increasing keratinized tissue. Compendium of Continuing Education. April 2015;36(4):pp290-297.

35) Atsumi et al. Methods to Assess Implant Stability: Current Status. International Journal of Maxillofacial Implants 2007;22:pp743-754.

36) Kotick et al. Abutment selection for Implant restorations. Inside dentistry July-August 2011.vol 7(7).

37) Abdou J et al. Rationale for use of CADCAM technology in Implant prosthesis. International Journal of Dentistry. March 2013:pp1-8.

38) Chee W. Impression techniques for Implant Dentistry. British Dental Journal 201(2016):pp429-432.

39) Bhakta S et al. Impressions in Implant dentistry. British Dental Journal 211(2011):pp361-367.

40) Hebel K et al. Cement retained versus Screw retained implant restorations. Achieving optimal occlusion and esthetics in dentistry. Journal of Prosthetic Dentistry 1997;77:pp28-35.

41) Assaf M et al. Screw retained crow restorations for single implants. A step by step Clinical guide. European Journal of Dentistry 2014. (Oct-Dec);8(4);pp563-570.

42) Chee E et al. Treatment planning of the edentulous mandible. British Dental Journal 201(2006):pp 337-347.

43) Zeynep O et al. Reconstruction of Edentulous maxillary and mandibular arches with implant supported fixed restorations using a digital treatment planning technique. A clinical Report. Journal of Oral Implantology 2008; 34(3): pp 161-168.

44) Thomason JM. Mandibular two implant supported overdentures as a first choice standard care for edentulous patients. The York Consensus Statement. British Dental Journal 207(2009):pp185-186.

45) Jivraj et al. Treatment planning the edentulous maxilla. British Dental Journal 201(2006):pp261-279.

46) Egilmez F et al. Implant Supported Hybrid prosthesis: conventional treatment method for borderline cases. European Journal of Dentistry 2015, July- September, 9(3): pp442-448.

47) Porter JA et al. Success and Failure of Dental Implants. A literature review with treatment considerations. General Dentistry 2005, Nov-Dec;53(6):pp423-432.

48) Yifat M et al. Characteristics of early versus late implant failures. A retrospective study. Journal of Oral and Maxillofacial surgery 2009(67): pp2649-2652.

49) Sudheer A et al. Dental Implant Failure: A review. European Journal of Biomedical and Pharmaceutical Sciences (2015);2(6): pp70-72.

50) Mahato N et al. Managing of Perimplantitis: A systematic review 2010-2015. March 2016.5:105)

51) Renvert S et al. Clinical approaches to treat peri implant mucositis and periimplantitis. Periodontology 2000; 168 (2015): pp369-404.

52) Prathapachandran J et al. Management of Periimplantitis. Dental Research Journal 2012. Sept-Oct;9(5): 516-521.

53) Geach WC et al. Osteointegrated Implant Fracture. Causes and Treatment. Journal of Oral Implantology 2011; 37(4): 499-503.

54) Bidra AS et al. Clinical guidelines for Recall and Maintenance patients with tooth borne and Implant borne restorations. Journal of ADA. Jan (2016);147(1):pp 67-74.

55) Todescan S et al. Guidance for the maintenance of care of dental implants. A clinical Review. Journal of Canadian Dental Association 2012;78:c107.

56) Palmer et al. Complications and Maintenance. British Dental Journal; vol 187(12) 1999:pp653-658.

57) Eswaran MA et al. Failure of Dental Implants, a literature review. International Journal of Biomedical Research 2015; 6(10):pp.756-762.

58) Elian et al. A simplified socket classification and repair technique. Pract.Proced.Aesthetic Dentistry 2007;19 (2):pp99-104.

59) Juodzbalys G, Wang HL, Sabalys G. Injury to Alveolar nerve during implant placement: A Literature review. J. of Oral Maxillofacial Research 2011, Jan-March;2(1): E1.

60) Chen ST, Beagle j, Jensen SJ, Chiapesco M et al. Consensus Statement and recommended clinical procedures regarding Surgical techniques. Int. Journal of Oral and Maxillofacial Implants 2009; 24:272-278.

61) Buser D, Chappius V, Belser UC, Chen S. Implant placement post extraction in esthetic tooth sites; when Immediate? When Early? and when Late? Periodontology 2000, 2017; 73: 84-102.

62) Malhotra N, Mala K, Acharya S. A Review of Root fractures: Diagnosis, treatment and Prognosis. Dental Update 2011 (Nov); 38(9): 615-616, 619-620.

63) Hedge M, Dahiya R, Shetty S. Horizontal root fractures, Diagnosis, Prevention and Management. A Review. Int. Journal of Medicine and Pharmaceutical Research 2013;1(4):367-375.

Printed in the United States
by Baker & Taylor Publisher Services